To my Olde Boot

we survived

I began writing this book many years ago, after witnessing the horrors of abuse in the long-term care facility where I was working. The manuscript was put on a shelf and occasionally dusted off to add another witnessed abuse. It wasn't until I was subjected to the debasing I received from my employer, the Saskatoon Health Region, Sask. Health and the Premier of Saskatchewan, did I decide to bring this book to fruition. It was not a labour of love neither was it a labour of hate. It is a book of fact, of truth. One cannot love abuse or cruelty, and one cannot live on hate; but truth is one thing I could, and do, live for.

There are countless people I would like to thank, not for input in this book for this was a singular project. The first person to make my list of thanks is my son who was responsible for editing my rough manuscript. He took that manuscript, turned it upside down and back to front to make it more readable, more palatable. And of that, I am most grateful. He rightly shares his name on the front cover.

I am also extremely grateful for the NDP leader, Cam Broten's Aide de Camp for her unconditional support. Her emails and telephone calls kept my spirits alive and carried me through what would become a living hell.

I am also grateful for all the support by mail, email and telephone calls I received throughout my ordeal. I recall being in a grocery store when a stranger came up to me, shook my hand and thanked me for coming forward and, as he put it, spilling the beans. It is these moments that made my journey more pleasant.

When one is under the gun one must tread very carefully. Thus, a couple of things were sidelined. One was a cessation of all social media. With our reliance on it, it proved a difficult task. The other was the inability to contact a good friend of mine. Dot is in a little piece of my heart, the part that holds good friendship. It was considered dangerous to communicate with her. Purposefully I decided to avoid any contact.

To my union, the SIEU West, I owe a debt of gratitude. Their guidance and professionalism were second to none. They stood firm and continued to reassure me from those that were brutally antagonising me.

Rarely do media find thanks. But I do with gusto for these people went out of their way to print and broadcast fair and unbiased account of my run in with the Heath care system. Dave Fraser of the Leader-Post is singled out for thanks for just keeping in touch. A simple phone call or email with, "how are things going," meant so much to someone being crushed by the weight of adversity.

The reader may wish to find out more about this case from the media perspective. Writing my name in any online search bar should bring up all articles that were printed. Television news can also be accessed. The Independent Office of the Privacy Commission likewise can be accessed for the report on my challenge of the government's release of my private and confidential information.

In the text, I have cited my sources and I extend my thanks. I have also cited SHRA policies and procedures. All cited sources can be found online and accessed free of charge.

It's been a long two years since I went public with my stories of abuse. I have always maintained I spoke the truth. No matter how many times I was asked, the story always remained the same.

Therefore, with the production of this book I can truly say;

Veritas liberavit me (*the truth has set me free*)

© Peter Bowden 2017

Cover picture courtesy shutterstock. Used under license.

TABLE OF CONTENTS

Time line of events	5
The big old Teddy Bear	8
Facility	17
Empty halls	23
Calamum vindictam prurit	27
Also starring	30
Purre	38
Let the inquisition begin	44
The gag	53
Office of the ambudsman	59
The fall guy	64
Into the breach	69
The ulcer	77
The catylist	85
The drinker	91
Slam dunk	100
The BM	111
Hypothermia, the silent killer	122
Always short staffed	126
The ulcer, again	133
The wanderer	140
The fall girl	148
The political storm	158
I smelled a rat, a political rat	162
The little old lady	183
The facts ma'am, just the facts	202
Abuse, how do we know	207
The numbers	216
The surveys	220

The next to last word	223
Life goes on	224
See me	228

TIME LINE OF EVENTS

March 2015	Cam Broten (opposition leader) raises issues of short staffing as a nursing home.
March 24	Email sent to Cam Broten explaining short staffing and abuse at my place of employ.
March 26	Meeting with management re: short staffing and abuse.
March 30	Information of short staffing and abuse released Via media interview and through legislature. Initial contact with NDP Aide de Camp.
April 01	Placed on day shift at work
April 16	2:00pm: phone call from management placing me on paid suspension. 4:00pm. Received allegations of impropriety via Email from Union
April 20	Private and confidential information illegally released to premieres office. Timeline: 10:34am From my employer to Ministry of Health 10:36am From Ministry of Health to the deputy minister's office. 10:42am From the deputy minister's office to the health ministers office. 10:52am From and unidentified staff person in the health ministers' office to the premieres office. 12:01pm-1:38pm many Emails sent to media via premieres Chief of Operations and Communications.

April 21	Premiere released my private and confidential information in the legislature. Informed house I had been suspended.
April 22	Media believed I had been suspended due to my whistleblowing. 11:00am meeting scheduled between employer and myself cancelled.
April 24	Letter to Office of Idependent Privacy Commission' First meeting between health region lead investigator and myself.
April 25	Discovery no whistleblower existed.
April 27	8:30am meeting with Saskatchewan Ombudsman. 10:00am. Informed by reporter of incorrect information Emailed to him. 11:00am Premeire challenged on information. Wlaked away from daily scrum.
May 22	Second investigation meeting.
June 2	Third investigation meeting
June 21	Fourth and last investigation meeting.
August 13	Terminated from my employer
August 17	Report released from Privacy Commissioner. 2:00pm Verbal apology from the premiere.
August 27	Written apology from CEO of Saskatoon Health Region Authority.
September 17	Wtitten apology from ministry of health.
January 18/06	Litigation against Sask. Health, Saskatoon Regional Health Authority and my employer commenced.
June 16/06	Settlement reached between all parties. Litigation and arbitration discharged

THE BIG OLD TEDDY BEAR

I probably identified this man with my youth more than any other person I had ever met. There was a photograph of him wearing a Canadian Navy uniform. He was standing behind a desk that contained several shooting medals and trophies. Surrounding him were several other Navy personnel. Some were dressed in ratings uniforms, others in officer uniforms. All were dressed in the old-style clothing of the Canadian Navy. A blue denim collar, surrounded by three stripes, stood proudly on his six feet five-inch body. It was perhaps the most recognisable item of his uniform.

It is often considered lucky to touch a sailor's collar. The bell-bottom pants were designed so that they could be rolled up easily when scrubbing the decks. Ratings used to have either five or seven horizontal creases. Unlike the stories of folklore, this did not represent the seven seas or five oceans but depended on the length of the sailor's leg. I remember my father telling me that when he was a rating, he would fold up his trousers into seven creases then lay them under his canvas sling. It got the job done, and he didn't have to send it to the Chinese laundry people on board ship to be pressed.

A white lanyard around his neck was originally used to fire the cannon on board ship. Later, a sailor would carry his knife with it.

In the encased photograph, my resident was the tallest of all. A broad smile revealed intense pride. He was a sharpshooter, a professional. I understood him instantaneously. It was unfortunate, but I never did find out what medals or trophies he had won. The photograph itself was nestled in a glass case deep-seated in the wall outside his room. All the resident's rooms had one. They were called history boxes. In them, the family could put a few items that represented the resident's past. One resident had his Doctorate in Psychology credentials in his case. One even had his first pair of tiny leather shoes. In another his first million-dollar year real estate sales certificate. And although we call them history boxes, almost to a one, dementia residents forget their past. What lay within the boxes become meaningless, forgotten times. These history boxes would sometimes keep me company at night.

In the case of my sharpshooter, on the bottom shelf of the history box was a small plastic model of a World War One Dreadnaught (the largest battleship built). Also in the case was a marriage photograph; both he and his wife were dressed in Navy uniform. I would often have to unlock the case and set the photograph back up as careless people would bump the wall, knocking the picture flat on its back.

If I hadn't known the picture was taken at a Canadian shooting range, I would have thought it was taken at Bisley, England. It is here that the world's best sharpshooters, military and civilian, meet every year. As in the photograph, camaraderie was critical in team success. Individual competitions showed prowess and skills. It was an honour to be designated the champion shot with a Lee-Enfield Mark IV 303 rifle. A bullet through a four-foot bull at 1500 yards was no mean feat. Other challenges involved the Smith and Weston 38 calibre handgun and the Sterling sub-machine gun.

My father was a superior marksman in the Royal Navy. He had been to Bisley many times. I well remember him returning home with medals and trophies and, what we all waited for, cash winnings. One successful year he became a member of the Queens Navy Eight, the eight best shots in the Royal Navy. Before the competition, the rifle range became his second home.

His favourite gun was the Stirling Sub Machine gun. His other favoured gun was the Smith and Wesson 38. Someone he knew in the shooting fraternity had made him a fitted pistol grip. It was made of African rosewood and was well known to the custodian of guns on the Navy shooting range. It was my father's pride and joy.

There was a certain satisfaction among this small group of men. No matter where my father sailed, and he sailed far and wide, some of the Commonwealth countries would put on a shooting competition. The aircraft carrier HMS Hermes (he was serving as Chief gunnery instructor, Petty Officer) ported in Kenya. Not only did the Kenyans put on a shooting competition for the gunnery crew of the Hermes, but they also treated them to a safari.

And so, as I assisted the resident with his care I felt a unique connection. I could talk his language. My resident had been a Petty Officer. Every time we met (he wandered a lot at night) I used to salute and call him Chief. I valued our relationship even though I had more than a suspicion he didn't understand me. But it was communication, and that to me was important.

He was a big fellow. The last time I checked his chart my resident weighed in at over 240 pounds. Height, 6'4". He was slow, slothful and he shuffled his feet. It was his disease. Not only had his memory been lost but his ability to walk. Speech had also been lost although hearing was still intact.

Very slowly we would walk hand in hand to the dining room. Although I gave him a cup of coffee each time he was up that early, rarely did he drink it. He preferred to walk about until he found a comfortable chair in the television lounge. There he was happy to fall back to sleep again. He reminded me of a giant teddy bear.

As soft and cuddly as he appeared, he would often fight like a bull when he was being dressed for the day. Often socks seemed to be the trigger for violence. I can only surmise he could not properly see the Care Aide putting them on his feet and this was, perhaps, the cause. However, there was no other way to put them on. We had to bend in front of him. We got to know the look on his face or the twinge in his muscles or even the grumble in his voice to know he was upset. At that point, both my partner and I moved away from him, well out of hitting range.

Tee shirts were also a problem. He did not like his head covered, and to put a tee shirt on him, it had to go over his head. As I got to understand him, I realised that everything we did for him had to be slowly explained before we acted. It took nearly a year before I can honestly say it was relatively safe to dress him.

If we had complex issues with him in the morning, then at night it would be more of an arduous task, a task that would injure me. He did not like to be wet. He would unceremoniously remove his saturated night pad and drop it on the floor in his room. He would then remove his nightgown or clothing if he were put to bed fully dressed. The toilet was not part of his psyche. Urinating on the floor would become his nightly routine. Often it would occur two to three times a night. The floor mop was always ready to go to work.

Working hard with the information I had gathered, I deduced the problem was at the staff level and staff on the evening shift. The resident wore pull up underwear during the day. Staff found it easier to toilet him. One night I found him wearing this type of pad. It wasn't wet, but I knew by 2:00 am it would be. I found an insert, which is a very thick liner specially designed for the type of incontinence product he was wearing. When he woke up and was wet, I changed his pull-up and added the insert. I also managed to get him into a dry nightgown. For the remainder of the shift, he slept like a baby, the first time.

I always considered assisting the residents to find a restful sleep as one of my important roles. I told the evening shift what I had done and the results I achieved. I had also ordered a pack of these pull-ups and inserts. I asked the evening crew to dress him in these incontinent products when putting him to bed.

For the next two weeks, the evening shift complied with my request. For those two weeks, the resident had an excellent sleep. Indeed, often he did not wake up at all at night. The experiment bore fruit, for when we worked with him to get him dressed he was more than manageable. It was almost a delight to finish my shift with a happier and contented resident.

Urinating on the floor had become a thing of the past. Striking out at the Care Aides trying to dress him became history, although it would not last long. Another advantage was no more back breaking exercise at night. Although ambulatory, when he did get out of bed, it would be 2:00 am, something I could virtually set my watch too. I was, of course, on my own at that time. I would not see my partner for another hour or more. It was up to me to get him back to bed; after all, if he fully awoke then he would not go back to bed but rather walk the hallways visiting other, still sleeping, residents.

I could not allow him to disrupt others; they needed their sleep. One way or another, I had to get him back to bed. I would change him then, per the dictates of TLR (turning, lifting, repositioning): I would sit him on his bed, raising it to my waist height. I was always loath to do this as I was on my own and there was a significant risk of the resident falling from that height. I would then raise the head of his bed to a ninety-degree angle. At this point, I should have been holding onto his back and under his legs to swing him into his bed. The problem was he refused to assist me. He was a dead weight. A 240-pound brick. He didn't move any part of his body. Indeed, as I tried to turn him, he fought me by holding onto the edge of the bed.

Every night it became the same performance, and every night I felt my lower back being abused. I could do nothing. As explained prior, putting my resident back to bed was not an emergency. I would have no assistance until my partner arrived. I was instructed to leave him wandering. And as much as I tried to explain that he would constantly walk into other resident's rooms, my complaints fell on deaf ears. And so when I found the answer to his sleep, I, and my sore back were overjoyed.

Day staff had told me that the giant of a man was more of a big teddy bear during the day. And of course, there was a bonus to all our efforts; he was more complacent with other residents.

Even though all the charting and information passed on to the evening shift, things not only went back to the way they were but became appreciably worse. For some strange, idiotic reason, not only did this shift give the giant a full night pad, the type with sticky tabs in each corner, but they did not put in an insert. It took less than four hours for my resident to return to his old confused self.

I raised the issue with the RN. I broached the evening crew with the problems I was facing and the excellent results I had achieved. For some unknown reason, I was ignored. The positive results, the improved quality of sleep, the more complacent during the day not to mention the lower stress on my back. It all seemed for nought.

It was a monumental frustration for me; I couldn't help but wonder why they would do something so asinine to a resident. He should never have faced that kind of emotional torture. And as much as I tried, I could not stop the stupidity of it. Unfortunately, he wasn't the only one. Two other residents faced the same indignation. Being put in a full night brief instead of a pull up would be the primary cause of one resident falling.

The term abuse not only occurs to residents but, in this case, to staff as well.

At some point in my career, I came under investigation. During one meeting, on hearing about my gentle giant of a resident and the fighting we had to endure, the investigator asked if I employed GPA (gentle persuasion approach). Of course, he knew I had taken the program. After all, he was aware of every license, diploma, certificate and course I had taken. The GPA was a 7.5-hour program. It was designed to assist Care Aides in being proactive and responsive to potentially violent situations. It was intended to give us sufficient information and guidance to effectively work in an environment with residents who have Alzheimer's disease and various other forms of dementia.

With our gentle giant being in the middle-third stage of dementia, gentle persuasion meant getting out the way of his dead aim fist. No amount of gentle persuasion helped. He was always ready for us, and likewise, we were ready for him. Our reaction was to leave him until he calmed down. If he failed to calm, then we would leave him in the clothes he was wearing.

Fighting to get him into his clothes seemed ridiculous at times. Violence served no purpose. If we couldn't settle him, then we would leave him alone. We would give it five to ten minutes before we would go back into his room and try again. It was not uncommon for me to return for the next shift with the resident still in the previous night's clothes.

One morning this gentle giant became like an angry wild elephant. To work with him was becoming impossible. His violence superseded anything I had seen before. Something was clearly wrong. While sitting on his bed he had managed to lay a punch on me, and it was a good one. He also attempted to punch my partner but managed only to graze her. She was behind him at the time. Like lightning he turned, firing a fist at her. I was holding on to his leg putting on a sock when I sensed him tense up. I shouted, "Look out!" She started to move back and away from him. His fist connected with her chest but did no more than push her further away from him. I asked if she was alright. She was shaken but not hurt. We left him to his devices.

The next day he was equally obnoxious. I looked at his chart. He hadn't had a bowel movement for ten days. I was told that staff would not give him a suppository. They were too frightened of him. The Care Aides and LPN would much prefer to see him suffer than to give him the medication needed. The day shift LPN informed me that he was receiving an oral laxative and prune juice. She felt that this was more than sufficient for his care. I questioned the length of time it had been since his last BM and the possible health consequences. A shrug of her shoulders and "I'm not going to have my staff injured over such an issue" was the ill-gotten reply.

I was confused. I had always assumed nurses were there to ease pain and suffering. I was fast learning that this is not necessarily the case. The possible health consequences for my resident were far reaching. Bowel impaction was my first thought. The second was a twisted bowel.

I wouldn't have given either medical emergency any thought except I had come across both in my time. In each case, the resident had gone at least nine days without a bowel movement. Both had been sent to the hospital. Both never returned.

During one of my interrogations, I was called to task in regards to my resident not having a bowel movement for those many days. Specifically, I was asked why I considered this abuse. I answered in the best way I could. "To allow someone to go for that many days without a BM was, in my opinion, unconscionable. It was dangerous and potentially deadly. And the LPN should have known better."

The investigator had sought the advice of a psychiatrist. I thought it strange. A psychiatrist usually doesn't get involved in internal medicine. On the issue of anger, however, it was his speciality, and he thought he understood the violence the resident was expressing. The investigator had sought the professional advice of the physician. The letter, mailed to the investigator, clearly stated that in his opinion any resident in late third stage dementia would exhibit the signs and symptoms we were witnessing. He concluded that violence was a known factor in the later stages of the disease. He gave no bearing on the fact that the resident had not had a BM in ten days.

I scratched my head. I had been the principle night-time caregiver for this resident for almost four years. I was aware of his peculiarities, his likes, and dislikes. I understood him and could communicate with him. I also understood the progression of his disease and the time's violence would rear its ugly head, and for no apparent reason.

"That morning I wasn't seeing signs of late-stage dementia for god's sakes! "I leant over to the investigator and looked beyond his sandy-pink rimmed glasses and into his eyes. "I was seeing a resident plugged with shit! If you had not gone to the bathroom for ten days, I imagine you would be more than a little miserable. And when it comes to the doctor? Anyone can reach to a shelf, draw on a medical book and come up with a predetermination of signs presented. Let me at the doctor, and I think I can quickly change his mind, don't you?"

The last time I saw the big old teddy bear was April 7, 2015. He looked just the same. I held out my right hand and shook his, then I saluted him. On April 16, 2015. I was suspended with pay. I never saw him again, and a little piece of my heart had been lost.

THE FACILITY

It all started mid-summer 2014. At that time, I was working as a Continuing Care Aide (CCA) in Saskatoon. The Long-Term Care (LTC) facility was new; only three and a half years old. It had eighty-nine beds on three floors. Each room was similar in layout. The spacious room afforded staff more mobility and ease of movement with their residents. It was a far cry from the old building that still stood and was being used for fifty Long Term Care residents.

I came to dislike this old part of the home. Its official name is South Wing although it became better known as the fifty-bed unit. The unit was antiquated, small and never designed for the type of residents now living there. Originally the old building had been used for those that could walk but needed a little extra attention. Perhaps they had difficulty finding the dining room or possibly the bathroom. Almost certainly they needed nursing services to ensure they took their medicine on time. The rooms and building were meant for a more leisurely, friendly time.

As with most old buildings, it had outgrown its original purpose. It was now housing level four plus residents, residents confined to wheelchairs and other restrictive devices. It had a small dementia unit where escape was all but impossible. It would be unfair to say that it was like a prison. Residents could walk and mingle, and they certainly were not confined to their rooms. But like the new unit, they could not leave without supervision.

It was a smelly place; stale urine and faeces permeated the walls and ceiling. It was a combined pollution of fresh air impregnated by odious vapours of human waste. This was the work I was involved in, and I took it all in stride, irrespective of how I felt.

Most staff on South Wing complained of being overworked, something that was a chronic problem. One of the few aides that still communicated with me explained that when she started working in Long Term Care, most residents in the nursing home were level two and three. She explained that most residents had the ability to help themselves and looked to the aide more for support than actual hands on assistance.

Lifting residents from their bed to a wheelchair was a rarity and then only as a means to an end. In those days, she explained, Care Aides would lift residents by themselves. Turning and repositioning were also performed by one person. It was an easier life. Staff were not rushed off their feet. There was more time to spend with residents. Talking, playing cards, singing along with musical guests. A few Care Aides spent their smoke breaks with residents. However, as time passed, all that quiescent, deliberate care slowly filtered away. Camaraderie with residents had shifted. Time was becoming scarcer. Also, more residents were arriving needing level four care. The elderly was living longer. The healthcare system was not ready.

Level 1 supports people with basic care needs

Level 2 supports people with low-level care needs

Level 3 supports people with intermediate care needs

Level 4 supports people with high-level care needs.

Lacking sufficient support at home, level two and three residents took up lodging in private (for profit) care homes. As their care became more demanding, they were transferred to Long Term Care facilities.

Strokes, multiple sclerosis, and dementia drove residents to nursing homes. Traumatic brain injuries, quadriplegia due to injury along with a host of medical conditions were but a few of the conditions we saw. However, wars had left many with chronic health conditions. Many had what we now know as PTSD (Post Traumatic Stress Syndrome). Police officers, firefighters, and ambulance attendants are starting to realise that their emotional struggles are related to their employment.

It is no wonder that nursing homes are filling up, and fast. I well remember one resident who served in World War II as a corporal. He was attached to the Canadian War Graves Detachment. When the battle was finished and the guns silenced, he would enter the battlefield. His job was to retrieve the dead. He would identify the deceased and place the body into a shallow grave for the short term. After the battle (won or lost) his detachment would then retrieve the bodies and transfer them to a war graves cemetery.

Not only was it exhausting work but it was also a mental strain on him and others like him. It would be an emotional trauma that would surface later in life. Whilst the following two statements are from the Great War (1914-1918), I believe it holds well for the brave men in the Canadian War Graves Detachment in the Second World WarExhumation companies comprised squads of 32 men. Each squad was supplied with "two pairs of rubber gloves, two shovels, stakes to mark the location of graves found, canvas and rope to tie up remains, stretchers, cresol (a poisonous colourless isomeric phenol) and wire cutters. A stake was placed where remains were found.

Experience was the only method of knowing where to dig. Indeed, the IWGC noted: "Unless previously experienced men are employed...80% of the bodies which remain to be picked up would never be found. Indications of remains included:

i Rifles or stakes protruding from the ground, bearing helmets or equipment; ii. Partial remains or equipment on the surface or protruding from the ground; iii. Rat holes - often small bones or pieces of equipment would be brought to the surface by the rats; iv. Discolouration of grass, earth or water - grass was often a vivid bluish-green with broader blades where bodies were buried, while earth and water turned a greenish black or grey colour.

It is piteous work this collecting of dead...after three or four days in the forward area too, it tries the nerves and causes a curious kind of irritability which was quite infectious - all the party being cross and out of temper, and it was quite easy to find oneself heatedly arguing some trivial point for no apparent reason.

It was no wonder then that our WWII resident would scream and pull his bed to pieces. We would find the screen to his window ripped from its mounts. One day he cracked the safety glass in his room, the window leading to the outside street. He would remove all his clothing. Rarely did he leave his room.

While the resident was on his deathbed, his daughter confided in me that he was the same while he was at home. It was something of the war that would not leave him. He was a haunted man. And yet he lived a quiet life, raising a family. It wasn't until after being diagnosed with Alzheimer's did the nightmare of his WWII years began to manifest itself.

She told me a story of her father being sent to fetch a body that was spotted in a pond somewhere in the European theatre. Her father and his buddy arrived at the pond, which had frozen over. They could see nothing untoward, so her father scurried down the slight embankment to the edge of the water. He used the butt of his rifle to crack the thin ice. Like a cork from a champagne bottle, a headless, mangled corpse popped through the opening. And just like a fish on the line pulling, the body bounced up and down waiting to be hauled in.

The shock of the corpse breaking through the small aperture in ice frightened him. Quickly, and without thought, he scurried on his buttocks up the embankment to join his buddy.

It is these constant reminders of things past that drive people to do outlandish things without thought. It becomes a chore for Care Aides to attempt to understand this type of resident and to help control their urge to destroy things.

So, it was those that who had gone to war became more populous in Long Term Care facilities. But then we also had those who had suffered the trauma of post-war life. Many women had worked during the war years not only for their country but for the money. Extra income meant independence, material things. They could do things never dreamed of. Independence was a major step. Dances with departing soldiers were common. Parties with workmates, their money to spend. It was a new lifestyle. But it was to come crashing down and quickly. When their spouses returned home, the women found themselves back to their nurturing side. Making babies, cooking meals, taking care of the house and, of course, the garden. Most would fret over the reversal of sudden freedom.

Smoking became a social standard. Cigarettes were cheap to buy and were plentiful. No one could have imagined the true cost of smoking not only on the arteries in the brain but other vital parts of the body. Smoking over a long period can (and often does) cause arteriosclerosis (hardening of the arteries). When occurring in the brain, the artery can neither expand nor contract. When a thrombosis (blood clot) loosens and breaks free of an artery, it can enter the brain. There it almost certainly will block off blood supply to a portion of the brain – a stroke. Depending on the size of the blockage a major stroke may occur. Paralysis usually results.

However, these blood clots may be so small only minute parts of the brain are affected. It is called a transient ischemic attack (TIA). It is a brief interruption of blood flow to part of the brain that causes temporary stroke-like symptoms. This is something often seen in the dementia unit.

Another casualty of war was the influence of cheap and easily accessible liquor. It is yet another product that causes hardening of the arteries. It can also cause thickening in the valves of the heart and destruction of the liver.

Dementia is not curable. The resident arriving in the unit will have on average two to three years of life remaining. Their quality of life will slowly diminish. They will forget who they are, where they are, why they are there. They will forget family members and even their spouse. In the end, they will have forgotten life itself.

Understanding resident's history is equally important to the knowledge of their care. But when someone who has learned all this valuable history of residents and understood their mood triggers is asked to leave the unit then something has gone horribly wrong. That is what happened to me. That is what happened to the residents I cared for.

EMPTY HALLS

TLR (turning, lifting re-positioning), is a system of Occupational Health and Safety (OHS) rules designed to aid the worker in moving residents/patients with the least amount of stress on the body. It is the law. So serious is the problem of back injuries to healthcare workers, a team of OHS by-law officers have been charged with travelling the province ensuring healthcare workers were complying with the Act. If a worker is found not to be complying with the rigid enforceable standards, then fines are levied.

There were two main reasons why this part of the Act was so rigidly enforced. The first, and most obvious, was that a number of personal injury claims were skyrocketing. It was putting pressure on the employer-sponsored insurance plan, the Workers Compensation Board (WCB). But it was also causing major increases in employer premiums. The more injuries, the higher the premiums. This reflected on healthcare budgets.

Budgetary restraints meant that extra workers could not be employed. And as we were short staffed at night when proper TLR protocols were required, there was insufficient staff to comply with the protocols, to do the work as it should have been done. Injury would occur.

On night shift our collective verbal missive was always the same. "Give us the staff, and we'll comply with the Act". However, it wasn't that easy.

All staff were required to be trained in TLR. The training had to be updated and on a continuing basis. This was a giant step in reducing injuries. However, rules seemed to be written by obscure people in equally obscure offices. Despite meaning well, the rules often don't reflect reality.

The new building employed most of the modern conveniences not found in many older facilities. Track lifts replaced the older medi-man lifts. This apparatus was most responsible for back injuries when picking people up from floors. It became the primary cause of back injuries. It was designed to lift someone from their bed, not from the floor. The lift bar would only drop to within three feet of the floor. If TLR trainers knew this danger, then nothing was done about it for several years.

The process for using this mechanical lift was like all lifts except having to physically lift the resident to attach them to the sling bar. Staff would apply the sling around the fallen residents, sit him up and then lift him the three feet so the sling could be attached to the lift bar. It was often a gruelling exercise, especially when trying to lift a 200-pound person. It was against TLR. It was a back breaker.

TLR is specifically designed to avoid injury through lowering risk. Often, through short staffing, implementation of the lift required any number of unique of ways to circumnavigate the rules. Often a resident was found fallen and in an awkward position. Legs under the bed, body in front of the toilet with legs under the sink, etc. Such positions would not be the exception but rather the norm.

To ensure no one could see what we were doing, we would close the resident's door. It was stupid really. Who was going to witness what we were doing, especially as it usually happened halfway through the night? But the fear of the TLR police, as the by-law officers were affectionately known, was so great, hiding what we were doing seemed natural.

Manipulating the resident was usually done by bending over and pushing or pulling him/her to a clear area. We could then attach the sling and manoeuvre the lift to a better position to complete the lift. I'm reasonably sure that had the TLR police caught us, we would have faced steep fines. For a Care Aide, they would have been $240.00; a

Supervisor (RN or manager) $400.00 and management, if it could be proven that training for staff had not been carried out, $1,000.00. (memo provided by management)

During day and evening shifts there are trainers/instructors on hand to answer questions or give advice when staff run into difficulty. At night, we did not have the luxury of that resource. We had to figure out any difficulties encountered by ourselves. It often resulted in weird and delightfully funny ways of lifting residents. It wouldn't be difficult to address the problem. Train a few full-time night staff to TLR instructor level, and the difficulty would be solved. But this is night shift. That elusive team of ne'er-do-wells whose skills are never questioned...and should be.

To comply with the TLR regulations, we had a fifteen-minute in-service perhaps once every two to three months. There was a questionnaire that went along with the tactile education. These in-services started at the beginning of our shift. On one occasion, the instructor took a little longer. Thus, I arrived at the dementia unit at 11:15 pm. I arrived alone. Not uncommonly, I did not have a partner that night. Thus, we would once again be working short.

Except for residents, the place was empty, ghostlike, eerie. There were no Care Aides on the unit. They had all left, gone home. I searched for the nurse (LPN). Likewise, she had gone home. The residents were alone, abandoned. Disbelief raised its ugly head.

When a nurse deserts or neglects a patient with whom he or she has an established provider-patient relationship without making reasonable arrangements for continuation of care and without reasonable notice, that nurse may stand accused of patient abandonment. In other words, once the nurse receives reports on residents, that resident is that nurse's responsibility -- until she passes the report to another nurse or until the resident has been transferred or discharged. (NSO)

This rule also applies to Care Aides. They too cannot leave their posts until they have been replaced. It was a serious breach of protocol. It was dangerous. Residents could have suffered the consequences.

When the night nurse arrived to give the night report, I told her of the incident. Her reaction was of genuine surprise. She couldn't understand her opposite doing what she did. The LPN was known to be a micro-manager. A person who rules by decree, and rules by the rules. I was questioned. Did I get it wrong? Was she with a resident, or perhaps in the bathroom?

I told her that the LPN's scooter was gone from the parking lot. I then added that I had toured the unit, finding all residents' doors closed. The Care Aide's coats were gone, and their work shoes were where they should be. "Nope!" I told my nurse, "they were all gone."

After a few minutes of disagreeable discussion about the situation, the RN shrugged her shoulders and told me that there was not much she could do about it. "It seems to me'" I said glumly, "that it's a case of who cares."I kept the knowledge of wrongdoing quiet, as did the nurse. As far as I'm aware no one else in the building that night knew of the situation. And as far as I know the night nurse did not do her duty in reporting the situation to management. It would become a pattern of deceit that would permeate the nursing home.

The reckless abandoners continued to work oblivious (or perhaps fully aware) of their guilt. It was a case of:

Hear no evil.
   See no evil,
      Speak no evil.

CALAMUS VINDICTAM PRUIT
(*My pen itches revenge*)

So what! I blew the whistle on elder abuse. Who cares? Not many, by all accounts. And although the press had a field day for a couple of runs, it wasn't until the government stepped up to the plate, releasing unsubstantiated rumours of my supposed violations of Health Region policies, that the media took hold of the story and ran a mile with it.

The media smelled a rat. They thought conspiracy. They had that instinctive hunch that something was wrong. Why would the Premier of one of Canada's provinces be so laisser-faire as to walk into a political storm without first ensuring his feet were on stable ground? Did the Premier believe he had the right to personally attack a whistleblower? Did he think that the public would believe him about my supposed indiscretions?

The media had something they could latch onto, and they did so with verve and gusto. They were adept at putting two and two together. During those few weeks, the Premier's ears must have been burning. His accusations were unfounded, unproven, false. And yet he stood in the House and spewed out his abhorrent lies without ever once looking for that truth.

In its summation, the report from the Office of the Independent Privacy Commissioner found the Premier should have concerned himself more with finding out the facts of the abuse as presented and not attacking the whistleblower.

There is no doubt the Premier set out to destroy a whistleblower. And in that, he was very successful. But then he was not the only villain in the story, not the only by far. Given that I worked at the Long-Term Care facility, I must assume a certain amount of guilt for the maltreatment of the residents. And if I am culpable then so is the staff that worked with me. Equally, because management was warned of this abusive behaviour many months before my coming forward, then they too must be drawn into the net of denunciation. All of this was explained in my email to the leader of the opposition. And yet we mustn't stop there. That would be too easy, for many would escape the brutality of truth. The Health Region had been informed of my scandalmongering and had worked to cover up the mess, and it was becoming chaotic. But the pool of malice only grew larger: in the wings was Saskatchewan Health and their political ties to the government.

The pot was full to overflowing. Everyone seemed determined to kill the messenger, the one who was speaking out for better treatment of demented residences. For <u>my</u> demented residents. All they wanted was a decent ending to their tortured lives. Despite proof of maltreatment, nothing was done to correct matters. The problem was no one gave a damn.

Even with proof staring him in the eyes, the Health Region investigator apparently found no mistreatment of residents. Or at least, that's what I assume for I have not, and will not, have the privilege of reading his report, ever, even though it's about me. He did, however, find the testaments of supposed wrongdoing given by myself to be accurate and demonstrating a neglect in care. As the investigation ended, it was obvious the investigator had listened to his masters. My reputation had been damaged beyond repair. Both the union rep and I saw the entire four-month process as a total misrepresentation of the truth.

During my termination meeting (which was revoked almost a year later), I stated to the two people sitting opposite me that what I had gone through was nothing more than a kangaroo court. I was determined I would not be silenced. All my corridors had been darkened. I did not have the inability to fight back, or so I thought. However, a small, but not insignificant light shone through the darkness that defeat brings. My Union had decided to try for arbitration.

That spirit drove me on to seek redemption from the three levels of care that had decided, arbitrarily, to destroy my working life: my employer; the Health Region; and Saskatchewan Health. They could have listened collectively to my complaints. They could have sought the truth, to correct matters. Everyone would have walked away wiser. All problems would have been satisfactorily and peacefully resolved. Instead, they brought out the knives.

But then, I know:

Veritas liberabit me (the truth shall set me free).

ALSO STARRING...

Working in a Long-Term Care Facility, sometimes referred to as nursing homes, is not unlike being in a play or a movie. A list of characters play out their individual roles, each one pivotal in the health and safety of the residents in their care. Remove any one character, and the entire story begins to collapse. Allow any one character to rebel, and once again the entire collaborative entity fails.

To understand the complexity of a Long-Term Care Facility is to enter a minefield of complicated roles and relationships. Each appears to have an ostensible desire to outshine and outperform one another. It has the sense of management run amok. It is within this myriad of performances that I found myself entrapped.

Who are these characters? What do they do? How do they relate to one another? Let's start somewhere near the top.

The C.E.O. The Chief Executive Officer, an extraordinary character whose role is never quite understood. In this facility, he is never seen. He is heard only when necessary and only if something has gone disastrously wrong. He is an expert at delegating. He prefers that his subordinates respond to their departmental difficulties. It's his Fiefdom, and he likes to rule with an iron fist.

His responsibilities should include but are not limited to: directing the operations of the facility; providing a plethora of services; providing programmes; overseeing staff budgets; establishing relations with other organisations and other management functions. It's not a job for the weak. Neither is it a job for a bully. Our CEO tends to hide in his office and only pops out to show he is alive. Night shift sees him, on average, never.

The D.O.C. The Director of Care. This person is most often seen by day staff. Night shift rarely, if ever, sees her. Her responsibilities are, to a degree: Supervising and reviewing nursing staff; overseeing resident care; overseeing department budgets; reporting to the CEO; maintaining a high standard of care; managing resident data and medical records and interacting with doctors, residents and family members. It is a difficult job one that takes a certain degree of tenacity. Our DOC attempts to compromise with staff. And by and large, she is successful.

The A.D.O.C. The Assistant Director of Care. To assist the daily functions of the DOC and to assume DOC duties when that person is away. Various tasks are assigned to this person. One is to maintain a professional contact with staff. Another is to issue memo's that are pinned on unit bulletin boards. Some concern Management/Nursing relations, others, new procedures for care. Some have the correct spelling but very poor grammar. Others have the opposite. Another is to visit each nursing unit during her shift to ensure continuity of care. Our ADOC is not particularly amiable. She is an antagonist. She is not ready and willing to compromise.

The R.N. The Registered Nurse. Most understand the RN as the person we see in a hospital. That concept is rapidly dying. We now see either an LPN or, most likely, a Care Aide. Upper management has determined that the role of the RN in Long Term Care is more administrative in nature. Indeed, it has been documented that the RN will spend up to 20% of her time performing administrative work. She is also responsible for dictating work requirements to staff under her supervisory wing. She also ensures that the work has been completed and that medical standards have been kept. Her nursing skills will be brought to bear when an accident or illness occurs, or someone is in need of treatment. Her role is varied, her responsibilities wide-ranging, her skills essential. Our permanent RN rarely listens to her staff. She never truly understands her role and is quick to complain and condemn without action. She is also somewhat unhurried and often complains about her workload

The L.P.N. The Licensed Practical Nurse. This person is the nurse most likely seen in a Long-Term Care Facility. Her training, while not as comprehensive as an RN's, is more than sufficient to practice in Long Term Care. The LPN is responsible for a nursing unit. However, occasionally at night, they may have to play the role of RN, especially if the RN phones in sick. When this happens, our LPN becomes angry, impatient, and complains to his subordinates that he must do all the work. Our LPN is not as intelligent as the RN. Both dislike one another. When the RN is on duty, he calls for her only when he finds his nursing skills inadequate. He shoots from the hip without first thinking about his actions.

The C.C.A. The Continuing Care Aide. They play a supportive role to both the LPN and the RN. Their main responsibilities lie with the residents. They assume the role of primary caregiver to their residents. They act as a liaison between the residents, the LPN, the RN, and family members, with the full-time CCA's having intimate knowledge of residents. This information is shared with other staff. Depending on its sensitivity, it may be withheld from family. Our CCA's have a tendency not to tell the truth. In their huddles, they speak their language and concoct lies. They are hard workers, but they are also lazy. Quickly getting work done so they can sit down or sleep seems to be their primary goal. Those CCA's who do not speak another language do the same. But they are more discrete.

The CCA is aware of the needs and wants of their resident. They do whatever is needed to fulfil their obligations. It is, without a doubt, the most underestimated accomplishment a caregiver can achieve. Their job is difficult. The CCA is rarely recognised as an intelligent creature. Indeed they will be shown to be imbecilic, stupid, and ignorant, and management will agree. Their superiors continually question their skills. "Micro-managed" is a term often used to describe their work environment.

The CCA is responsible to her superiors. Then that ladder of authority or, as some see it, the line of domination, comes into play: the LPN, the RN, the ADOC, the DOC, the CEO and the Board of Directors. Of course, we must not forget the Health Region with their glut of management. Continuing Care Aides are also responsible for the residents and the residents loved ones. Their role is the most difficult of all. They are there when a resident is admitted to the unit. They will be there when the resident dies. Until then they will become friends with their residents and their families. The day the resident passes, the CCA will work a normal shift. Unless it is their day off, they are not allowed time to attend the funeral. CCA's are the workhorse of the facility. However, they are the most ignored.

The INVESTIGATOR. He is the lead investigator. Apparently, there are a few investigators under his wing. He is employed by the Health Region. My employer is affiliated with that Health Region. His job is to apply the administrative law to an investigation. The application of administrative law is called the 'balance of probabilities.' The 'balance of probabilities' test asks: "is it more likely than not that something happened?" The test is also referred to as '50% plus a feather.'

He will look at all the aspects of all the allegations, the ones that claim I was abusive, and the ones that imply misconduct. He will apply the law to his conclusion. He will not seek the truth; he will seek anything but the truth. He will go on a witch-hunt. His job will be to protect my employer and conversely the Health Region from the stigma of abuse in Long Term Care. He will appear to be a nice man, genuine and caring. But he will become a bully and will refuse to answer any of my questions.

After twenty hours of interrogation, he will provide a report that only a scant few will ever see. I will not be one of them.

Rt. Honourable Brad Wall MLA. The Premier of Saskatchewan,

He is the Premier of the province of Saskatchewan. His role will be to stand in the Legislative Assembly and state that all health care workers would be protected if they came forward with complaints. He will stand behind the Privacy Act and say the information -- my private and confidential information -- given in the House and to the media was for the public good.

He will not acknowledge that there may be some truth behind the abuse allegations. He will not ask Saskatchewan Health, the Health Region or my employer to consider the allegations. His primary role is to destroy the whistleblower. He will act like anything but a Premier. The Premier will eventually and publicly apologise to the whistleblower. He will become known as Bad Brad.

Rt. Honourable Dustin Duncan MLA. Heath Minister. He is a true and faithful servant to his Premier and the Saskatchewan Party. Whatever his Premier states he will repeat without question. It will be repeated in the House at question period and in the media scrum. The truth will be stretched very thin. He will try to make everyone believe that the Saskatchewan Party has spent a significant amount of money in Long Term Care. He will also try to make people believe that more than adequate staff have been hired in care homes to cover worker shortage. He will tell people that twelve million dollars allocated to Long Term Care in the previous budget were sufficient.

Cathy Young. Saskatchewan Party Communications Director.

She will be the catalyst for all things bad for the whistleblower. She will pass on incorrect information to the Premier from emails she received. Those emails will come from my employer to the Health Region and through Saskatchewan Health to her office. She will email members of the media so they can inform the public. She will not ask if the emails are true.

The Rt. Honourable Cam Broten MLA. The leader of the Official Opposition. The New Democratic Party. He will receive an email from the whistleblower. The email will explain my working conditions on the night shift. He will raise the issue in the Saskatchewan Legislature. It will be comforting to him to have the first person working in the health care field come forward with a legitimate complaint. He will bring to the attention of the people of Saskatchewan the plight of their health care system. After the whistleblower is terminated, he will ignore him. It is strange how politicians and their staff disavow someone as soon as they run into problems. Perhaps I had become useless to them, no longer having juicy information for them to use. Perhaps they saw that I was a liability to their cause. Whatever the case it's a classic whistleblower's dilemma.

The finger of fault is all too common an occurrence. Those that stand on the bottom rung of the ladder of success, such as CCA's, seem to receive the brunt of "It's his fault." I have never seen a Registered Nurse terminated. Likewise, Licensed Practical Nurses seem to have an impervious job security.

However, I have witnessed an Assistant Director of Care being 'let go.' It's a more pleasant term than terminated, fired, chopped or sacked. Apparently, she was not of the calibre my employer was looking for, even though she had been in her position for over a year and had an excellent rapport with the staff.

All staff I talked to agreed it was a terrible, discrediting thing that happened to her. What I didn't know was that management had waited until she had lost all of her nursing seniority before terminating her. It was a painful blow. To get back to work she had to start at the bottom rung, so to speak. Although I knew her well (she allowed me to call her by a nickname), I didn't know the truth about her relationship with my employer for over three years.

There is no doubt she deserves my empathy. Management, I have learned, can be deceitful. They can look you in the eye and spin a good lie. Perhaps this was this ADOC's problem. She was just too damn honest. And I do miss working with her.

The Whistle Blown

After I had blown the whistle, I found myself in a den of traitors, turncoats and tellers of lies. During 2014, almost to a person, my colleagues agreed with my perception of negligence. They agreed on what I had seen and on what was being done -- or not being done, as the case may be -- to the residents.

They agreed that it was wrong. All the players became traitors to the cause. CCA's, LPN's, RN's, ADOC, DOC and yes, the top dog himself, the CEO. The Premier, the Minister of Health, the Saskatchewan Party Director of Communications and yes, the Health Region, also became traitors to my residents. Each appeared to conspire against me, to quieten the message, to suppress the truth. Any one of them could have listened, could have witnessed for themselves the cruelty the residents were suffering. They could have taken corrective action. Instead, they feigned that I was deceiving them.

I became the devil incarnate, a rogue, someone to spit on, kick at, to misinform the public about the truth, my truth. In their eyes, I was a charlatan, and they wanted to see me spend the rest of my life in purgatory.

Although everything in this book is true, I have avoided mentioning names. It was not a difficult decision to make. It has been done to protect the innocent. Although there are a plethora of guilty people, I have elected to keep their names obscured. There seems little point in destroying careers. One is enough. It is a fitting way to protect what little integrity they have left me.

I did not report the nurse to the SRNA (the Saskatchewan Registered Nurses Association) although I have accused her of some of the more horrendous crimes. Likewise, I did not report the LPN to SALPN (the Saskatchewan Association of Licensed Practical Nurses) even though she did something that was abhorrent to any human being, which will be presented later.

Even without names attached, those who performed unspeakable acts should hold themselves accountable. If they are espoused to Christendom, then perhaps they should give penance by flogging themselves.

Who am I? What is my pedigree? Where do I get my knowledge? Within my stable of close acquaintances are; psychiatrists; anaesthesiologists; many RN's; several LPN's; medical nursing assistants, recreational Technicians, Emergency Medical Technicians, etc.

As for me? I've been working as a Care Aide for eleven years, seven of those with people suffering dementia. I have worked almost exclusively night shifts for twenty-seven years. Eleven of those were spent as an Industrial EMT. I have taught Advanced First Aid/CPR for the Red Cross. I have also taught instructors how to teach.

As you turn the pages, a new world will open. Few have entered that world, and fewer still understand what happens there. In that strange land of twilight and silent voices, negligence and abuse occur. It is hidden by the dark cloak of night. It took my becoming a whistleblower to turn the light switch on and shout "this is wrong."

I believe that it is incumbent upon every person, politician and layman, to shout at the highest level:

Our elderly deserve better.

THE PUREE

"No more fucking food for you, you miserable prick!"

"That's right; you tell the bastard. No business putting up with that shit. We ain't paid enough to take this crap."

The speakers, two Care Aides, were assisting residents to eat their supper. The dining room was swollen with all the residents in the nursing home. It was a midsummer's evening. The facility was stuffy and hot. Humidity swirled in the air as kitchen chafers belched out steam keeping food hot. The building itself was old. It had very limited air conditioning. Even the hallways to residents rooms were equally as hot. The only solution to the excessive heat management provided was by placing several fans on each floor. They served little purpose than to move the stale hot air around.

In the stagnant, almost unbearable heat, people's nerves were ragged. The high temperature and the cacophony of cooking pans striking one another did not help matters. Severs calling out special orders made the situation unbearable. But it was the resident in question, the one at whom the tirade was directed, who would receive the brunt of the Care Aide's brutality.

Residents living in long-term care homes eat varying types of meals depending on their ability to swallow. There are three types of food served: ordinary food, the typical food found on the average family dining table; food that is ground up for those that have a limited ability to eat solid food; and puree for those that have great difficulty swallowing. The resident in question ate this third type of food. The resident being helped was exasperating. A year before he had suffered a severe stroke. Working with him became, to some, an irritant. But he was totally dependent on others. As Care Aides, our role was to look after his welfare whether that was emotional or physical. While he sat at the table, he could fully comprehend his whereabouts and what was happening to him and around him.

Although he was cognitive, he could not speak. His stroke had removed that ability. I could see that communication through his eyes was possible. It was a difficult process, and it did take time, but interrelationship was possible. The Care Aide responsible for the resident this evening either did not understand him or refused to converse with him. She had worked with him on dozens of occasions, so she certainly was aware of his ability to communicate.

The resident was sitting at the dinner table in his Broda chair, a chair that supports a resident's entire body while rendering them immovable. Dependency on others often causes depression. If he was ever depressed, we were unaware of it as he never showed that side to us.

This evening he appeared his same old self. As he sat in his chair with his head resting on the pillow, he coughed several times. There was phlegm in his upper airway, but his ability to cough deeply enough to get it out was impossible. His stroke had robbed him of that as well.

The resident smelled. His body odour was rank due to oozing bedsores (ulcers). Even though these ulcers had dressings applied to them that morning, a purulent discharge managed to flow through the gauze. The nauseating smell permeated the air surrounding his table. Evidently, the Care Aide was not happy. But there seemed an underlying issue to cause her annoyance. I would find that out a little later.

The resident sat in a roomful of knives and forks clattering on plates. He sat with one other resident waiting for his food. Because of his stroke, he had difficulty swallowing. It is easy for someone with his condition to aspirate their food. Therefore, care is needed when assisting him to eat.

The dangers of a stroke victim eating are thus described:

When solids or liquids that should be swallowed into the stomach are instead breathed into the respiratory system, or when substances from the outside environment are accidentally breathed into the lungs.

This condition can cause aspiration pneumonia. The highest risk of this condition is seen in older adults with a history of:
- lung disease
- seizure
- stroke
- dental problems
- needing help eating
- swallowing dysfunction
- impaired mental status
- neurologic diseases
- People at any age can have certain additional risk factors. People with additional risk factors include those with:
- a swallowing dysfunction who cough during meals or have difficulty breathing

a history of vomiting a severe chronic illness that prevents them from chewing properly(Gale Encyclopedia of Medicine)

The resident had several risk factors. He had had a stroke, had dental problems, needed help eating, had a swallowing dysfunction that caused him to cough during meals and a severe chronic illness that prevented him from chewing properly.

He needed a high protein diet to assist in healing his ulcers. A body without food or the wrong type of food heals slowly. Without adequate and proper foods death often arrives more quickly.

There is no doubt the Care Aide should have been on her guard. She should have been watching for warning signs of aspiration. Care Aides are purposefully trained to assist residents with their food. There is a standard of practice subscribed by all Diploma Care Aides. There is a prescribed method of assisting someone eating pureed food. Time and patience is the ideal environment. Delivering food to the resident should be done slowly and with purpose. A quarter of a teaspoonful should be the maximum amount offered at any one time. No food should be offered again until the resident's mouth has been emptied. It is equally important to watch the swallowing process.

The position the Care Aide found herself in was not unusual. Assisting a resident eating is among many of our daily chores. She had been a Care Aide for several years. Therefore, she should have been prepared mentally and physically for the task at hand.

She busied herself talking with another of her colleagues. They were both engaged in assisting residents with their meal. Attention to detail was negligible, as they both seemed to concentrate on talking to one another. Their conversation was full of small talk with plenty of laughter. Discussions about Management filtered in and out as she started to assist her resident with his meal. It was obvious to me she wanted to finish her chore at the same time her colleague finished hers. However, her colleague's resident could swallow reasonably well and would be finished in short order.

To speed things up, she decided to bend the rules. She elected to give her resident his food in heaping teaspoonfuls. He could not swallow fast enough so he 'pocketed' some of his food into his cheeks. For the second and third heaping teaspoonful, this worked. The more he ate, the faster his Care Aide fed him. She did not notice that he was not swallowing sufficiently to keep up with her. His cheeks became engorged with soft food. He began to choke.

The resident's face turned a bright red. Neck veins bulged, his eyes began to protrude, and he could not breathe.

To get air into his lungs, he opened his mouth. He began to drool his food. As it oozed out, he had a violent cough. The propulsion of food and air shot into the ether and rained down like sludge.

If his Care Aide had been watching her charge more closely, she could have avoided the obvious. But she wasn't. Talking to her colleague seemed more important at the time. She turned her head to see what the commotion was, her resident coughed violently once again. This time she took the full force of the rest of the food that had been in his mouth. Her uniform became saturated. She squealed as she pushed herself away from the table. She cleaned her face of some of the food, her eyes bright. She glared at the resident, upset and angry.

"No more fucking food for you, you miserable prick!" she yelled as she began wiping more of the food from her face and hair. Her colleague looked on wondering if she should laugh or sympathise. Sympathy won out.

"That's right; you tell the bastard. No business putting up with that shit. We ain't paid enough to take this crap."

Then the unthinkable happened. With all her might, the Care Aide pushed the chair away from the table and into a wall. As the chair hit the wall, the resident bounced around. He then started to slide down his chair, stopping when his knees hit the bottom of the chairs' table. He was in an extremely uncomfortable position. It was clear his ungainly posture was putting pressure on some of his deeper ulcers.

His upper torso was halfway down the back of the chair. His facial expression spoke volumes. He was hurting. But the Care Aide would have none of his obvious discomfort. After she had cleaned herself, she pushed him to an anteroom. There he would sit until the rest of the residents had finished their meal. It didn't matter to her that he could hear others eating and talking. He must have been hungry for he had eaten not even a mouthful. The Care Aide kept to her commitment. She did not give her charge any more food. So deep was her anger that at snack time she refused to give him anything. The resident did not eat again until the following morning.

Her rush to assist her resident to eat was as bizarre as the incident itself. Smoking was not allowed in any SRHA affiliates or their grounds. And as she was a smoker, and so to her colleague, she wanted to take her smoke break with her. But the other resident was eating much faster. Therefore, she tried to keep up by engorging her resident with his meal.

The resident not eating again for 16 hours was abuse. Add to that the way he was assisted being fed and was cursed at should be sufficient for some disciplinary action. However, if we add the way the resident was forcibly removed from the dining room all within sight and hearing of other residents was a calamity. And the fact he was sitting incorrectly in his chair, and in pain, and not being helped just added to the debacle.

After the incident both Care Aides went outside for their smoke break. Smoke breaks were not official breaks. They were intended to ease the trauma of not being able to smoke in the facility. Only if there was sufficient time could smoke breaks be taken

Clearly, this Care Aide put her resident's life in danger for the sake of a cigarette with her colleague. It is but one example of the oft' brutal life in a Long-Term Care Facility.

DEFINITION OF ABUSE

"A single, or repeated act, or lack of appropriate action, occurring within any relationship where there is an expectation of trust, which causes harm or distress to an older person;"
World Health Organization's definition of abuse.

THE INQUISITION BEGINS

Email from my Union representative:
Thank you for getting back to me. We will be meeting at Avord Tower on the 8th Floor. This is right by the Sheraton downtown. I will meet you on the main floor, and we can go up together. See you then.

It didn't take long for my union to answer my email. They had been made aware of the change of date and location of the meeting. It would take place in two days, on April 24, 2016, at Health Region (HR) lead investigator's office. It turned out that the time of the meeting had to be changed three times before we could sit down with him.

4:30 pm on a Friday afternoon seemed an odd time to conduct an interview over such a serious complaint. But then, I began to reason, my employer and SHR did not want any worse publicity than they had already received. At that time of day whatever news was generated would be too late for news deadlines. As far as I was aware, no reporters from either television or print media knew of the meeting. The entire exercise was cloaked in secrecy.

I met my union rep for the first time in the foyer of a downtown building. She was very pleasant and exceedingly knowledgeable. We sat for a good ten minutes while she explained the course of action we were about to embark on. It seemed daunting, but I had right on my side, and I would face whatever was directed at me with head held high.

I was over sixty-one years of age, only three and a half years from retirement. What, I thought, could they do to me? I could retire and go my merry way. True, I would have to find other work. But naively I thought Continuing Care Aide work was in abundance. I would find work with ease. I forgot how nasty people treated whistleblowers. How stupid I was.

My rep and I were shown into a small office. We were told that the investigator would be a few minutes. It was enough time for me to pick up a trinket from a side table, look at it, then break it. A good start, I thought as I lowered my shaking head.

The office itself was quite small. It had two small desks. On each desk was a computer monitor. Two chairs had been made available for my rep and I. Between us was a small round glass table, the table with the now broken trinket. On the wall behind us were framed university awards, one for a social work degree while the other held a congratulatory award for being a good investigator. I'm not sure what university was mentioned, but an American school of study does come to mind.

The office had one window that looked onto 21st street. If I stretched enough, I could catch a glimpse of the South Saskatchewan River. The junction of 21st Street and Fourth Avenue was in full view. The roads were busy, it was Friday afternoon, after all. A younger (and what I would discover), bombastic, bearish man barged into the office, his office. Following him was the proverbial winds of change. He introduced himself as the Health Region's chief investigator. Although pleasant, he tried to articulate his words carefully. It reminded me of a bumbling politician trying to give an unrehearsed speech. I was amused. Here was a Canadian trying to speak the quintessential Queens English and failing. I was reminded of Sir Winston Churchill's great oratory skills and his ability to carry people along on every word. And as much as he tried, this man couldn't.

His role, he explained, was to investigate the accusations of impropriety against me. He further stated that his role was neutral. He wanted to arrive at the truth. It was, therefore, important that I tell the truth. I butted in and forcefully. I told him that I had two reasons for being there. One was, to tell the truth. The other was to find the identity of the individual who was responsible for leaking my personal information to the government. "That information," I told him in no uncertain terms, "travelled from my employer through SHR to the government. A lot of other people and I would like to know the answer." I didn't know at the time how long it took for that information to travel from the bottom of the ladder to the top rung. Several months later I was to find out that it took mere minutes.

It was clear by his answer he was not interested in finding the source of the leak. His role was to investigate me. As far as I was concerned, however, the accusations I faced were a direct result of my whistleblowing. If that were to be proven, then he would be bound to investigate the complainants of abuse I had raised. After all, I surmised, this was where the whole tragedy started. He did not respond further.

It would be many months later that I found out my union was not interested in the abuse occurring at my employer's either. I was told they could not find a definitive link between the complaints against me and my whistleblowing. Further, to that, the union informed me should I introduce anything about the abuse at my arbitration hearing they would stop me. They obviously didn't want the issue raised. Perhaps they didn't care.

I had found that link. It had arrived two months into the investigation. But it didn't matter. No one seemed to take note. No one seemed to care. The thought of residents and their care being muted by an investigator who, by all accounts, gave the impression to he had been charged with the singular task of burying the whistleblower bothered me immensely.

My representative and I were informed that the investigator was certified in his craft. "My job," he said, "is an information gatherer. I make findings of fact." He made certain to add, "I have no vested interest in the outcome of this case." It turned out that his non-vested interest in the case would drag me into a world of deceit and lies. It would become a witch-hunt, one of his own, and his employers, my employers, devising. We believe his goal was to find guilt on my part.

He continued. "The Canadian test in administrative law is called the 'balance of probabilities'." He went on to explain: "the 'balance of probabilities' test asks: 'is it more likely than not that something happened?' The test is also referred to as *50% plus a feather*."

Why he said what he did still resonate with me for he added: "If you feel you have been harassed in this process you can contact the Provincial Occupational Health and Safety Office." Notwithstanding that little gem, he continued, "You have the right to exercise your legal rights available to you under the law. You have the right to appeal an eventual investigative decision via the collective bargaining agreement grievance process. (That appeal was eventually brought on by way of a grievance).

"Should my complaints fail the test as stipulated by you, is there an avenue for redress, an appeal outside of the Union?" I thought it a fair question. But as to *all* my challenges, he declined to answer.

Even at this early stage of the proceedings, I was becoming somewhat flustered. The man was conceited and pompous. Indeed, I thought him boorish. I began to have doubts that I would get a fair hearing.

He told me that I had the right to be provided reasons for his investigative decision. He also stated that that decision would probably be provided in written format after the investigation by Saskatoon

Health Region Authority Human Resources and by my employer. Whether he knew it or not, I would be stopped from reading his report by SHRA lawyers. As of March 2016, my union and their lawyers are still trying to reverse this SHRA decision.

At one point, and away from the hearing, he did mull over the possibility that there may not be a written decision. He thought that perhaps it would be delivered verbally. This, I thought, was inflammatory and I began to smell the possibility of a cover-up.

"After I'm comfortable that I've established an accurate/ reliable foundation of facts, I'll do my analytics and write a report, make findings, and then test my findings to policy, both your employer and Saskatoon Health Region Authority policy. I was informed that my employer had their respect and dignity policy. But in every other way, the nursing home adopted the Health Regions policies."

My employer had adopted all the SHRA policies. Although I had a reasonable idea this was the case; he was the first person to come forward and state it. It interested me. I could now search SHR policies on-line to determine his line of attack. And it would become an attack, a war of words, a deliberate debasing of my healthcare skills.

My rep asked the investigator: "When the final report is written do we get a copy of the report or some kind of executive summary? What do we receive in terms of a written decision?" What she said, I thought, was a critical question. His answer would force him to take the stand if litigation ever resulted.

He answered I thought sheepishly, making sure of his words. "The employer, consulting with the Director of Human Resources and even perhaps the Manager of Labour Relations of the Saskatoon Health Region, would make that determination". He noted that I would have the right to know why I would not be able to read the report. He then used his escape from what would become a controversial issue, "It's not my decision." It was a catchphrase, one that was often used during the investigation.

I snapped back with venom. "So, they become the judge and jury. My rights to a fair trial have been squashed."

I was to be judged by a Kangaroo court. And I wasn't going to win.

I was told that all accounts of allegations against me were written verbatim. It took a considerable amount of time and frustration for the investigator to explain what 'verbatim' meant. He explained that verbatim is a word-for-word account of the complaints submitted to management by employees. He went on to say that there would be typos in the text. He then dropped a mini-bombshell by saying that "he didn't change the verbatim complaints **very much.**"

I found it difficult to believe that Someone of Authority and in charge of legal documents would even consider altering them. He had been handling legal documents most of his working life. To alter them was not only immoral but almost certainly illegal. His only saving grace was if he highlighted the changes and applied his signature. He did neither. I was left wondering just how true all these accusations were. (All the allegations of impropriety were eventually withdrawn by my employer).

I was half way through my 61st year. The pressure in the room was tense, and I could sense he wanted this investigation over. He wanted to show his employer he was eminent at his craft. I, on the other hand, had something to prove. I was going to lose my job of that I was certain. And at my age, I would not have the enthusiasm or the time to start a new career. I was going to put up a fight. I didn't know how to fight. So, I took the battle one line of each accusation at a time.

"I believe the leak of my confidential information either came from my employer or your office," I said, a slight wavering showing my nervousness. I wanted to bring the case of whistleblowing back into the conversation. I thought it an important part of the investigation.

"Whatever the case I believe this investigation is bound by its terms to discover how the leak occurred. If I can find a positive link between being suspended and whistleblowing then, I believe, you are bound to investigate."

He stated categorically that the leak did not come from his office. A week before, on April 16, 2015, I had received the first rough draft of the allegations against me. Per the attached letter, an SHRA labour relations consultant would be carrying out the investigation. On April 22, 2015, this had been changed in favour of the SHRA lead investigator, the man I now sat before. The accusations had been in his office for at least eight days. There was speculation that his office may have been aware of them on or before April 11, 2015, although that is yet to be proven.

"We know the accusations have been in your office for eight days," I said, trying to keep my conspiracy theory alive. "They may have been in your office for up to thirteen days. Within SHRA I find it hard to believe it could be kept a secret."

All the television networks carried my story. Saskatchewan newspapers had also carried it. The Premier and the Minister of Health had verbally attacked me. They had received and publicly preached to the media information of which I was unaware. I still find it very difficult to believe that the investigator's office would sit on a file and no one would be privy to it, least of all me.

The meeting was over. I was given a copy of the accusations against me. Both my rep' and I used a separate meeting room to review them. The review was quick. The stench of hate from fellow colleagues began to waft from the pages.

If altering the documents wasn't sufficient, the investigator made me aware that he would bring into the investigation further improprieties that I may have executed. The paragraph reads: "On occasion, circumstances arise where allegations beyond the initial scope require probing. If scope is expanded, it will be done so at my discretion, and the dictates of natural justice applied." I would eventually face more than eighteen charges. In the last meeting, July 21, 2015, my union rep' charged him with soliciting. (January of 2017, I discovered soliciting did occur.)

His face turned red as he tried to fumble his way past that indictment. But he had been caught. Two charges four years previous had been laid against me. He claimed the information was given him voluntarily. I said nothing. It wasn't worth my time or effort. Disgust filled my very soul, and the investigation had yet to begin.

In the meeting room, I sat and pondered the silliness of it all. Most of the charges were frivolous and were not very exacting. I told my rep that many were symbolic. There were half-truths, innuendos and complete fabrications. My nervous smile covered the heartfelt sadness that was beginning to consume me.

I had rarely caused issues during my tenure as a Care Aide. I did receive a disciplinary letter years prior, and at a different facility. That was mainly due to health problems. Any disciplinary memo is supposed to be expunged from an employee's personal file after two years. That is entrenched in the SEIU contract with SHRA. Through digging through computer files, the investigator found that disciplinary letter and raised it in our final meeting. I was furious; my union rep was stunned. I now realised that SHRA and their chief investigator would stop at nothing to see my name and reputation purged from their collective souls.

The meeting ended with the appropriate courtesies. My union rep' and I left with my spirits dampened. But I felt a sense of relief. The original accusations against me were vague, one line, one sentence. The complete allegations received by management, and of which I received a copy, were more palatable. I could identify those that had filed the complaints. I now could date each one. It was less than a month between them all. My memory was good, very good. I would have all the answers for the investigator at our final meeting. I was determined to completely crush the lies and innuendoes that, by all accounts, were written in blood.

THE GAG

She was sitting in her Broda, anxious. Her Care Aides had just sat her down. As she was a total lift, the resident was vulnerable and counted on others for her care and mobility. A mechanical lift was used to remove her from her bed to her wheelchair. A mechanical lift comes in a variety of models; basically, it's a wide-based device, on wheels, with an overarching neck and a hanging set of arms to which one attaches a sling. The sling is attached to the resident, and the resident is attached to the lift. The lift operator, a Care Aide, raises the resident from the bed into a suspended sitting position, the sling providing a seat, not unlike a baby swing on a playground, albeit more malleable. The neck portion of the lift uses hydraulics to raise the resident, and then they are swung away from their bed and placed in a waiting wheelchair.

There is no question many elderly people are afraid of mechanical lifts. Many have a fear of falling. There have been many incidents of falls from these lifts. From frayed and broken slings to residents being put into slings incorrectly, it doesn't take much to cause harm to an elderly person.

This resident had fallen in the past, and the fear of falling again was part of her psyche. Her Care Aides should have known her history, should have known that she was fearful. But she was also tired. She had a condition called sleep apnea.

Sleep apnea is a common disorder in which you have one or more pauses in breathing or shallow breaths while you sleep

Breathing pauses can last from a few seconds to minutes. They may occur 30 times or more an hour. Typically, normal breathing then starts again, sometimes with a loud snort or choking sound.

Sleep apnea usually is a chronic (ongoing) condition that disrupts sleep. When normal breathing pauses or becomes shallow, the resident will often move out of deep sleep and into a light sleep.

As a result, the quality of sleep is poor. That lack of quality makes the resident tired during the day. Sleep apnea is a leading cause of excessive daytime sleepiness. This resident was no exception. Tiredness would haunt her throughout her day.

- Untreated sleep apnea can:
- Increase the risk of high blood pressure, heart attack, stroke, obesity, and diabetes
- Increase the risk of, or worsen, heart failure
- Make arrhythmias (ah-RITH-me-ahs), or irregular heartbeats, more likely Increase the chance of having work-related or driving accidents

CPAP (Continuous Positive Airway Pressure) appliance is the most common treatment for moderate to severe sleep apnea in adults. A CPAP machine uses a mask that fits over your mouth and nose, or just over your nose. The machine gently blows air into the resident's lungs. The pressure from the air assists in keeping the airway open while the resident sleeps. (National Institutes of Health).

By her bedside was a CPAP machine. It had not been used for a long time. I had been working in the facility for over three years, and I had never seen it in operation. It was not surprising that she was tired.

She used to scream when she was being helped to get up. Her neighbour also called out loudly when she was being helped to get up. Screaming or calling out when scared is not an unusual occurrence. But to the Care Aides this morning it was worse than an annoyance.

The resident's history showed she had had a severe stroke several years prior. It was this malady that brought her into the care home. Because of her condition, conversation with her was impossible. It was a matter of telling her what was being done. But over the course of time and due to the same morning routine, the Care Aides failed to talk to the woman. It was assumed she understood the daily procedure.

At 95 years, old memory is not always as sharp as it was. Many studies have shown that exercising the brain helps increase memory. In this case asking the resident questions would possibly help. It would certainly encourage her to become involved in her care. This minor adjustment in her care, slowing down, waiting for her to think about the question, might have helped.

Her room was small, barely large enough for her bed and the mechanical lift. A small sink along with a built-in wardrobe completed the ensemble. It was a difficult environment in which to work. But that was what Care Aides did, often making the best of what they had and often struggling. Swearing under one's breath was common. Swearing out loud was uncalled for and foolish. This Care Aide was more than foolish.

As she was being prepared for the lift, the resident became anxious. She began to scream, some would say uncontrollably. The Care Aide in charge acted. She wanted to stop the howling. She was at her wit's end. The room was small. She had difficulty manoeuvring between the bed, the lift, and the resident's Broda. The resident next door began to scream. The Aide had had enough.

Without thinking, or perhaps on purpose, the Care Aide stuffed a brown washcloth into the resident's mouth. It was wrong. It was abuse at its most shocking. But it did give her what she fought for, peace and quiet. She could continue her work with ease although her wild profanity continued, unabated.

In this facility, two different washcloths were used. A white one was used for face and hands and upper body. A brown cloth was used exclusively for peri-care or peritoneal care. The perineum is the area in front of the anus extending to the fourchette of the vulva in the female and the scrotum in the male. It is also described as the diamond-shaped area corresponding to the outlet of the pelvis, containing the anus and vulva or the roots of the penis.

For female residents, peritoneal care involves wiping the vagina from front to back, cleaning out the labia and vaginal opening. It also involves wiping the buttocks.

The brown cloth stayed in the resident's mouth until she was placed in her chair, though sometimes it stayed in place until the resident in the next room was up and ready for the day. It's unclear whether the cloth ever obstructed her breathing, although it is a possibility given that this was a typical morning ritual for the resident.

It is unknown if the brown cloth corkscrewed into the resident's mouth had been used on her that morning.

I had a chance to talk to this 95-year-old resident one long, sultry day. It was many months before she began screaming. She had been a Saskatchewan Registered Nurse. She told me that ever since leaving high school, she had practised her craft. She had been trained in Saskatoon and, when retired from the hustle and bustle of hospital nursing, she had settled on working in a Long-Term Care Facility, not unlike the one she was now staying in.

In her youth, she had been required to travel to aid sick people. As she talked I could only imagine her nursing during the thirties when money was short, jobs were few and far between and if you were lucky enough to have employment you did what you were told and without question.

Her mind raced back in time. In her fractured speech, I discovered that a doctor had instructed her to go and assist in a delivery of a baby at a farm. The farm was about twenty miles from town. To get there, she had to catch a bus to the nearest village and then walk the rest of the way. She never mentioned what time of year it was, but I held autumn in my mind. I had the impression it was during the drought in the thirties.

She told me that when she arrived, the farmer's wife was in an advanced stage of labour. She quickly set to work and helped the mother deliver her fourth child.

When mother and child were safe and comfortable, she set about reviewing the health of the remainder of the family. Satisfied all were as healthy as could be in those lean times she set about making a deserved meal for the family. It was part of the job. A nurse in those days did all the chores.

With a wry smile on her face, the old nurse then said that for eleven days she took care of the baby, mother and family. She did not hesitate to cook, clean, and wash clothes. While the mother was resting after the birth, the nurse did all the chores expected of a farmer's wife. Somehow when I said that nursing had sure changed, sorrow filled her voice. That, I'm sad to say, was the only time we had a conversation.

Whether the guilty Care Aide was terminated or allowed to resign remains an unanswered question. Whatever the answer this person popped up again several years after the event. Again, she was working as a Care Aide. Her demeanour had not changed, and I feared for any resident under her care.

How was she caught? Until 9:00 am the permanent bath Aide assisted her colleagues, getting residents ready for the day. She was in the room and witnessed the incident. A union shop steward was also present. Nothing was said.

It was the Saturday night shift following the incident when the duty night nurse and I heard the story. It fell like a bombshell. As horrific as it was, the Care Aide mentioned it in passing. A minor incident. Something that didn't need to be worried about.

When questioned, it became obvious the resident was scared not only of the perpetrator but all the Care Aides on day shift. There were bullies on staff that carried their aggressiveness with hate. It was a poisoned facility. Management was aware of the bullying but did little to stem the rot.

Had it not been for two hours of discussion, cajoling and direction, the story may never have come to light. But it did and kudos to that brave Care Aide who stood in front of management and said what she had to say. Was she protected from her colleagues? As far as I am aware no one ever suspected her of reporting her fellow Care Aide.

OFFICE OF THE OMBUDSMAN

My wife and I were invited to a meeting at the Saskatchewan Ombudsman's office in Saskatoon. I had emailed them, giving them the same detail as I had given Cam Broten about the ratio of Care Aides to residents that I (and my colleagues) had witnessed at our place of employment. They were very interested in what I had to say. My wife came along for moral support. She always did. The expression "my rock of Gibraltar" could not be attributed to a better person. She is a retired Registered Nurse who had spent almost her entire career in geriatric care. She understood the problems that I faced where I worked.

The Ombudsman's office had been busy with a directive from the government. They were charged with finding the truth behind allegations of improprieties in Long Term Care facilities. The government had been deeply harmed by the bad press. We were less than a year away from an election and, I believe, they needed the truth to come out early. Then they could bury it.

The lead in local newspapers and television had been sensational. A family had alleged abuse by a Care Aide in a care home. A loved one of theirs had lost a tremendous amount of weight over the previous few months. She also had many second- and third-stage ulcers on her back. It was clear most were caused by shearing, moving her without the aid of proper equipment.

The family asked all the appropriate questions. The answers either were not forthcoming or they made no sense. They asked questions of the Care Aides, nurses, management and even housekeeping. No one would, or could, provide an adequate response.

The resident's family decided to take matters into their own hands. Clandestinely they placed a hidden video camera in the room. They would find out what had happened and what was still happening. The video of maltreatment was substantial evidence of abuse. Released to the media, it took the government by storm. The government opposition had been frustrating the governing party over its failure to respond to the increasing crisis in Long Term Care.

The government took little time in ordering an inquiry. It seemed that this was the incentive for others to step forward with their horror stories.

In another incident, a Care Aide slapped a resident several times on the head. The resident was demented and did not have the ability to understand simple commands. Again, the family placed a hidden camera in the resident's room. It would not be long before the local constabulary charged a Care Aide with assault.

Although general neglect within the Long-Term Care facilities had been identified, it took the combined efforts of Cam Broten and the families of those mistreated for the government to stand up and take notice.

The Ombudsman took six months to investigate the Pandora's box of problems before issuing its report. They had discovered over thirty complaints of abuse. The independent office condemned the health care system and its care of the elderly. Shortage of staffing, shortage of funding and shortage of proper training led to the disastrous events as laid out in the final report.

Besides my wife and I there were two people in the room. Both had notepads and were writing an appreciable amount of information. I wondered why they were writing as I was also being recorded. I was told that this was standard practice. My curiosity satisfied, I continued dutifully answering their questions when, to my annoyance, my cell phone rang.

I was a little embarrassed and apologised for the interruption. It was close to 10:00 am. We had been answering questions for about one and a half hours. The investigators halted the proceedings so I could take the call. It was a reporter from the Regina Leader Post. He was one of the few people I got to know and trust. He told me that he had received an email from the Premier's Director of Communications. He wanted my reaction. "Reaction? Reaction to what?" I asked.

The email was damning. It contained information regarding serious allegations against me. One of those allegations spoke of sexual harassment. I was stunned. At first I didn't know what to say. My mind raced through every accusation levelled against me. Nowhere had I read any words of sexual harassment. At no time did either word exist. Was this a trap? Swallowing deep, I answered his question with honesty. But he wanted more. He wanted my permission to go to print. I couldn't let him do that, not yet.

The knives were out and were being sharpened. But this was more than a knife, it was a sword, and I felt it being aimed at my heart. I had to move very carefully, and yet I felt the urge to give my two cents worth to the Premier and his damnable cronies.

The reporter told me that on Thursday the House rose early, at 11:00 am. He wanted to challenge the Premier about the email during the press scrum. I told him he could do that. He seemed happy. That was the last I heard of it that day. However, the next morning I received an email from my contact within the NDP office. It explained what had happened and what should have happened.

Often government will send an FYI as "background" to reporters, and indicate so, meaning it shouldn't be reported but is their info. That is what (the Premier) was claiming the second email with a lot of detail was. (Leader-Post reporter) and others didn't believe it.

My understanding is that late morning Monday, (Premier's communication Director) sent the first email to four reporters or so.

One reporter (from Leader Post), replied and asked her how she knew this. It was in her reply that she said all the quotes that are now in the stories, about sexual assault and the like. They are claiming this email was background but did not indicate such in the email. The Premier is now also denying knowing it was sent and saying his communication director has been punished, but we know he was told what was in that email as early as the 23rd. I will forward those statements after this email.

The main point that still remains is that the Premier asked his communication director to send these emails and provide your personal record to reporters, it is on the record, this cannot be denied.

My contact then added a simple statement that has remained my constant companion since this all started.

This is all so stressful, sorry for what you have been through.

The next email, sent the same day, helped solidify, in my mind, the Premier's goal. He was out to bury the whistleblower any way he could. I quickly learned that there are no niceties in war.

Hey Peter,

Below is some detail on the amount of detail that was released in the second email by the Premier's director of communication. The Premier confirmed in the house today that the second email cited in the Leader Post article with all the information was sent to their reporter. They claim it was "background", but the reporter has said on the record, on CBC radio Friday, May 1st that he did not believe it was "background" at all.

How are you? I hope you're well. The legislature media scrum is always held in the rotunda, which is adjacent to the Legislative Assembly Chamber. Among those holding microphones and recording devices, two women stand to ensure every word is captured. They are not reporters. One works for the Saskatchewan Party, the other for the NDP. Both work in their respective communications office. It would be unthinkable for anything said by the leaders or their MLA's not to be recorded. Posterity is expensive.

I received a telephone call from my NDP contact. I was informed that the Thursday morning scrum had turned into bloodletting. The Premier had been peppered with questions regarding the explosive email. My contact seemed excited. She told me that she had never witnessed anything like it. The Premier had become so upset he left the scrum without answering any questions.

I had won a small victory.

For the rest of the day, the sun shone just a little brighter.

THE FALL GUY

He was found sitting on the floor of his room. His head was caught between the head rail and the bed frame. It took a mechanical lift, three Care Aides and a nurse to extricate him. The resident was in extreme danger. It was a case of abuse.

SRHA (Saskatoon Health Regional Authority) advises that all beds should be lowered to their lowest point when being occupied. This, we were told, is a measure of safety for the resident. Falls are common as residents attempt to get in or out of bed themselves. As of 2014, all Long-Term Care beds have had their bed rails removed to avoid entrapment. This case preceded this arbitrary rule.

There are several types of beds being used in nursing homes. The newer ones sink to within four inches of the floor. This bed is designed for residents who are likely to roll out of bed. Therefore, safety or fallout mats are provided on each side of the bed. Because the resident is almost certainly a lift then Ideally the bed should be placed in the middle of the room. This way both Care Aides can access each side of the bed.

Another type of bed stops about eighteen inches from the floor. This bed is usually given to those who are ambulatory (able to walk). The third type of bed comes to rest much higher off the floor. Bed-ridden residents are given this bed. This person does not move at night.

Whatever the bed used, staff are required to raise the bed before performing any care. A Caroll bed may take up to thirty seconds to reach the appropriate height, waist height. Therefore, resident care can take considerable time, time some people are not prepared to give.

This resident was immobile. He was bed-ridden. Ulcers (bed sores) were always lurking on a resident such as he. These wounds can cause major injuries. Treatments tend to be very expensive and often precipitate an accelerated death.

To help reduce ulcerating injuries, some residents were given air mattresses. This mattress was designed to reduce pressure on the body and especially the joint areas. It is at the bony prominences that these sores develop. To further reduce the risk of pressure points, this mattress had no baffles. The mattress had an inflation device at the foot of the bed. As soon as deflation was detected an air pump would engage bringing the mattress back to normal inflation. A mathematical formula was used for each resident using these mattresses. Residents state of health and weight were considered. However, what was not considered was a resident's ability to move.

This bed-ridden and immobile resident had a feeding tube attached to him. His condition was such that he needed turning every two hours. Any risk of bedsores was dealt with diligently.

My partner and I were aware that any movement of the resident was potentially dangerous. We had another resident on a similar air mattress and would often find her trapped against the side rail. It wasn't until I witnessed her moving at night did I begin to understand the problem.

The law of physics states that trapped air, under pressure, will move along the path of least resistance. Therefore, as the resident moved, the air underneath was pushed up and behind her. The more she was pushed away from the centre of the bed the more air would move to her side. The situation grew exponentially. Once started there was no stopping until the resident met a solid obstruction. As soon as she became wedged against the bed rail, all movement stopped.

She couldn't call out; she didn't have the ability. Besides, her head was often found in the downward position and being pushed onto the bed-frame. During rounds, she would be found entrapped. We would have to physically manhandle her back up and to the centre of the bed.

We always hoped it wouldn't happen again during the shift. All too often it did. Each time the situation occurred, it was duly reported to the duty nurse and recorded in the resident's chart. To my memory, I believe the resident lay on that mattress for many months before it was removed.

Knowing the history of these mattresses, we set our resident in the centre of the bed. We then blocked him with several pillows running along both sides of his body. His head was similarly blocked. We were satisfied that he could not unintentionally move. I then lowered the bed to its lowest point.

I elevated the head of the bed to an angle of 45 degrees. This was standard practice for residents with difficulty breathing. We then re-checked our work. We came away assured he was safe.

The nurse, an LPN, entered the room a short while later. Post investigation determined that a series of mistakes had been made. Those mistakes were alarming and were diametrically opposed to the rigorous training nurses are subjected to.

She needed to attach a new bag of feed to his feeding tube. It was a simple task. Remove the empty bag and attach the full one. The LPN raised the bed to her waist-level. She then lowered the side rail but left the head rail in its correct 'up' position. The feeding apparatus was on the opposite side of the bed. Instead of walking around the bed, the nurse leant over the resident to fix the new bag. In doing so, she moved a few of the pillows so she could reach the machinery. When done, she raised the head of the bed to 90 degrees. When questioned she said that it was to stop any regurgitation. She then pushed the loose pillows against the resident and left the room.

She had forgotten to lower the bed to its lowest point. She had also forgotten to raise the side rail. Furthermore, when she replaced the pillows, she merely pushed them against the resident and not jammed them against him.

The pillows on the left side of the resident stayed tightly in place. The right side had been slovenly replaced. The resident began to move. As pressure built up behind him, he moved faster to his side. The support pillows on his right side were pushed away. As the side rail was not in the 'up' position, he was forced out of bed and to the floor. He dropped about four feet to the Lino-covered concrete.

As the resident's body slipped to the floor, his head followed. It was at a 90-degree angle to his lower trunk and legs, so he slid down straight. As his upper torso hit the floor, his head snapped back and against the inside of the headrail. It became wedged.

When my partner and I arrived, he was turning blue (cyanosis). His breathing was impaired. He could not get enough oxygen to meet the body's demand. Death was a distinct possibility.

We quickly removed his head from the choking position. He soon pinked up (skin turned to normal colour) as oxygen once more began to circulate. We quickly lowered his bed, and he was placed back in it. We then raised his bed and jammed pillows on both sides of his body. His head was reset to 45 degrees. We were comfortable that our resident was once again safe.

Bound by conscience, I wrote a report about the incident and submitted it to the Director of Care. I cited all the problems and submitted a rational plan to avoid a similar accident. One of my conclusions was to stop using the potentially dangerous air mattresses. I became aware that, through my report, air mattresses were immediately banned in Long Term Care Facilities.

Through all the horrendous mistakes the nurse made, nothing, as far as I'm aware, was ever done to bring her to task. Indeed, the next night she was back at work as if nothing untoward had happened.

It appeared as if residents had become second-class citizens. Their health and welfare became secondary to that of employment of staff. It was more important to keep what staff management had, irrespective of quality, rather than try to replace someone.

The resident received care well below the standards expected of an LPN. The Director of Care failed in her duty to bring this nurse to task. Had this been but one incident in my four years there as a Care Aide then perhaps, just perhaps, I would not have mentioned it. But this nurse had a running problem related to standards of care, from leaving the medication room door open to leaving the nursing home without staff coverage so she could have a cigarette.

I would find out that she was not alone in the small club of night nurses who, by the very nature of their willingness to work nights, lowered the accepted standards of care.

INTO THE BREACH

On April 30, 2015, I received an email from the investigator. He told me that the scope of his investigation had been expanded. He would be looking into the care of residents where I worked. He asked me if there were any specific residents that I believed were being abused. As requested, I supplied the investigator with a list of those I felt should be investigated.

On May 1, 2015, I responded with the list requested. In it, I identified seven cases of what I considered to be abused residents. I also explained why I thought they should be on such a list.

On May 5, 2015, the investigator emailed me asking for further clarification:

He asked for the identification of the RN and the LPN on duty the nights I claimed abuse was occurring. He also asked for the names of colleagues that could verify my information. He then asked what type of abuse I felt they were suffering from, listing several: physical, psychological, systemic, sexual, medical, abandonment, neglect, human rights, financial.

And then the silly questions started. Did I know if the resident's family members knew of the alleged abuse? Did the resident's doctors have concerns about the suspected abuse? Did I make my employer's management know of my concerns? When did I make them aware?

On May 6, 2015, I responded with the following email:

In the summer of 2014, I informed our R.N. that residents needed turning before 0400. I specifically identified one resident as a top priority as a reddened area on her hips were no longer blanching, and that skin breakthrough was imminent. The RN told me, and in no uncertain terms, that no resident needed turning in the entire building except one as she had MS (multiple sclerosis). Because she was cognitive, she would quickly become uncomfortable.

The R.N. repeated herself the following night shift. Her statement angered me. I believed that dementia residents became equally uncomfortable, especially lying in one position for at least six hours. To a one, all night staff knew I was extremely upset at the seemingly uncaring attitude of the R.N. I had made it very clear to anyone who would listen that I would not stay at the nursing home if this were the attitude of the senior staff. I began my search for different employment at another SHRA Long Term Care facility. When I calmed down, I decided I could not accept the nurse's ruling and began to break TLR rules by turning and changing residents by myself. I continued to change/turn residents by myself until December 16th of 2014.

As per the investigator's request, I then went about identifying the types of abuse.

Skin breakdown was a strong probability due to residents not being changed or turned and being left in pads soaked in urine. I then quoted from the Mayo Clinic:

Bedsores are caused by pressure against the skin that limits blood flow to the skin and nearby tissues. Other factors related to limited mobility can make the skin vulnerable to damage and contribute to the development of pressure sores. Three primary contributing factors are:

Sustained pressure. When skin and the underlying tissues is trapped between bone and a surface such as a wheelchair or a bed, the pressure may be greater than the pressure of the blood flowing in the tiny vessels (capillaries) that deliver oxygen and other nutrients to tissues. Without these essential nutrients, skin cells and tissues are damaged and may eventually die. This kind of pressure tends to happen in areas that aren't well padded with muscle or fat and that lie over a bone, such as spine, tailbone, shoulder blades, hips, heels and elbows.

Excess moisture or dryness. Skin that is moist from sweat or lack of bladder control is more likely to be injured and increases the friction between the skin and clothing or bedding. Very dry skin increases friction as well.

Bowel incontinence. Bacteria from faecal matter can cause serious local infections and lead to life-threatening infections affecting the whole body.

Residents who could not move should be turned at least every two hours. It was well known within the medical community that this would help in reducing skin damage (ulcers). I firmly believe the RN was complicit in the abuse/neglect of residents by allowing physical/medical situations to occur when they could, and should, have been stopped.

I then answered what I thought was a silly question. Due to working night shift I have no knowledge of whether members of the family or the resident's physician had any knowledge of my concerns. However, had either taken the time to read the resident's progress notes they would have seen my report on the matter.

The only way I could treat this resident was to turn her every two hours. I did not have a partner at the time, so I went ahead and performed the duty on my own. True, I broke the rules. True, I could have been disciplined. But according to Saskatoon Health Region's TLR regulations, it would have been very difficult to terminate my employment.

When asked if I could identify the date I could only estimate that I first informed the RN in mid- to late summer of 2014. However, we followed SHR's policy of charting by exception. Therefore, after two almost identical inclusions in the resident's chart, no other mention was made. I went so far as to photograph the damaged area of the resident's skin and showed them to the RN. It made no difference. As far as I know, she did not look at the resident's skin condition. I had used a skin integrity chart showing images and text of the stages of ulceration. With this information, I had identified the areas affected as being in stage one skin breakdown. There was no doubt in my mind that the resident's hips were nearing stage two, the stage where the skin is open to infection. One test is to press on the centre of the reddened area. The area should return to its original colour and quite quickly. However, in this case, the area pressed stayed white, a condition known as blanching; blood was not returning to the compressed site. She also had significant skin discoloration on the outside of her feet on the bony prominences. Her right ear also became troublesome with it often becoming reddened due to pressure.

The night RN received an email from management. She told her staff that our fall statistics were too high and that we were to call any fall that was close to the residents bed a slide out. Although the bed was only four inches from the floor, TLR stated that falling to any height lower than the previous height was a fall. I challenged the RN about the decision. She reiterated the information from the email directive. From then on, any resident that fell from bed was categorised as a slide-out. Therefore, no documentation was done other than a brief note in a resident's progress note that the resident had slid out of bed.

We surmised that the new fall reporting was due to our response to the plethora of falls that had transpired previously. On one such night shift, we recorded five falls on dementia alone. It was a given that there would be one fall per shift.

Should such a fall happen, the nurse, as well as another staff member, would have to attend the resident. The RN would ask the usual: "Are you hurt anywhere?" before lifting the resident back to bed using a full mechanical lift. The RN would then fill out a fall-report, which would then be transferred into a resident fall program on the computer. This report would then wind its way through the plethora of wires and silicone chips to a central data bank at SHRA. Each month a chart was released to all SHRA affiliates showing the data that had been collected. Management, we understood, was not happy with their placing.

As the new rules were put in place, the RN informed staff on dementia that they need not call her if it were a simple slide-out. If there were obvious signs of trauma, then that would be a different matter. It was left to unqualified staff to perform assessments on fallen residents. No one appeared to be upset. What part-time and casual staff thought about it I have no idea. But whatever the case, it was wrong, ethically and professionally. However, nothing was done, no one cared.

All slide-outs were recorded in resident's charts. Other than a verbal exchange between night and day shift, any slide-out vanished into the ether.

One resident did fall, and far from her bed. Not only did she not have a fall-out mat, but she was known to be ambulatory and could toilet herself at night. Thus, when we received an alarm that she was out of bed, we gave her several extra minutes before we would check on her. I believed residents should have as much autonomy as possible. Toileting is a private matter, and I always tried to provide that little bit of comfort.

When I arrived at her room, I found the resident approximately ten feet from her bed. She was adjacent to her bathroom and sitting on the floor. This was a classic fall. The resident had tried to walk to the bathroom; however, she had urinated on the floor instead and had slipped in it. I found her with her right leg tucked underneath her buttocks and her left leg stretched out. She was holding herself in a sitting position using both arms. I contacted the RN. I also contacted my partner. We would have to use a full lift. As luck would have it, the room came equipped with a ceiling track. Lifting the resident would be quick and easy.

Knowing the mentality of the nurse, I quickly informed her that this was a fall. She said nothing but went about her duties. As usual, she asked the resident if she was hurting. The resident failed to respond. As if silence was golden we were instructed to lift her and get her back to bed. As the RN left, she said that we were to chart this as a slide-out. It was a falsehood, a deception, and I would have nothing to do with the fabrication. I was not about to see my reputation tarnished. This scenario had transpired twice before, and I had gone along with the same instructions from the nurse. But not this time.

I did not see a fall report generated by the nurse, which was usually left on the office desk for me to fill out my part. I decided that I would enter the fall information, although in brief, in the resident's charts. This, I believed, would impart me from any blame should injury occur to our resident.

On the afternoon of March 25, 2015, I received a telephone call from the DOC. She informed me that I would be transferred to another unit that night shift. Aware of my dislike of any unit except dementia, she was quick to point out that the move was not intended as punishment. It was, she stated, with respect to the other staff who rotated to other units every sixty days. She also stated that other staff members were complaining that I stayed in one place.

I thought it strange that the second sentence of the phone call mentioned punishment. It was a known fact that the way management got rid of staff they had issues with was to change that employee's shift schedule. My wife and I read between the lines. I felt that I was on the hit list.

That evening, after checking my blood pressure several times and finding it very high, I phoned in sick. I would not go to work until things had been resolved. Both management and I had agreed to a meeting the next afternoon.

It would be a tense meeting. It was held in the ADOC's office with the DOC in attendance. At 2:00 pm the meeting started. I handed the ADOC a sick note from my doctor. She leant over her desk and accused my doctor of falsifying the sick note so that I would avoid working in the other unit.

I was angry. My respect for the medical profession and all those that work in it runs deep. My respect for my family physician was tantamount. How dare a simpleton ADOC, who was an LPN to boot, suggest my doctor would commit such a breach of protocol? With my dander up, I reached across the table and tapped the document, explaining what the injury was.

I had been in Havana, Cuba the year before and had taken a nasty tumble on the sidewalk. The end of my left humerus (upper arm bone) had been chipped away. Although painful, my physician had monitored it closely. It had been decided that the body would probably absorb the small piece of bone and that surgery was not necessary. However, a year later that elbow and its opposite were causing me severe pain. I was sent to an imaging centre. The radiologist had found both elbows had minor osteoarthritis with the bone chip still lodged in the left elbow. I challenged both managers to phone the radiologist and discuss the results.

My annoyance calmed. We got on with the meeting. I informed both managers of my assertion that abuse was happening in dementia. I told both that at least seven residents were on the list. I explained, in detail, what was happening and why. We were understaffed, I told them, and I was left on my own for up to four hours each shift. I informed them that the night RN was aware of my concerns but took little if any, notice of them. Further, I explained that many residents needed turning to avoid the risk of skin damage. The ADOC stated that none of the 139 residents needed turning as there was no skin damage. At that point, I knew I was beating my head against a brick wall. The

RN and now the ADOC were saying something remarkably similar. No one needed the professional standard of care that was demanded in Long Term Care.

The remainder of the meeting subsided into a communal think tank on how to reduce the issue of short staffing without adding extra staff. To my amazement, one idea that I had to alleviate the issue bore fruit. I was told that both managers would look seriously at my proposal, run it past the other night staff and even ask the union for their blessing.

The meeting ended with a, "Are you going to be at work tonight?" The DOC then added, "We will have a nurse that can do most of the heavy lifting. She knows the unit very well. She's worked there for several years. You'll be okay. You won't have to lift" Stupidly I agreed to work. My sick note indicated that I should not 'push, pull or lift anything heavier than 5 kilogrammes. Both managers thought that their solution to manning the shift was more than workable. How wrong they were.

THE ULCER

Staff had been informed that the new resident had requested a transfer to the Long-Term Care Home where I was working. It was not an unusual request. People like to make choices; this was his. We had an empty bed, and we made the room ready for him. The bed was placed close to the window, and the nurse and I placed several chairs in the large room as we expected family members to be with him. We made sure there was sufficient place for the gurney to be positioned by his bed. There was a fully equipped bathroom, but we both agreed that if he were in the later stage of decline, he would not be using it.

Information by telephone from his previous nursing home suggested he had very little time left. Death was just around the corner. He wanted the transfer because many years prior his wife had died at our nursing home. It was a family belief that should he die where his wife did then their souls would meet in heaven. It was his unabashed belief that she would be waiting for him.

The resident arrived late that evening. Evening staff had gone home. The night shift took responsibility for the incoming resident. When transferred from one facility to the next the resident is accompanied by nurse-to-nurse transfer documents. This information would include a family doctor, medications, history of falls, skin condition, etc. The accompanying resident's charts would hold his long-term history and would be reviewed later. The transfer papers reported nothing unusual. Our new resident was not eating or drinking. We gave him ice chips to quench thirst. There was nothing to indicate anything more than that the resident was facing death. The writing was scratchy. A fine point pen had been used. But it was how the relevant information was written that caught my eye. It looked hurried as if time was running out.

Perhaps the ambulance had arrived early, and the nurse had not had time to finish the paperwork. Perhaps she had an emergency of her own. Whatever the case, in the section for existing skin condition, nothing had been written.

Both the nurse and I followed the resident down the long hallway. He was wrapped in blankets and strapped to an ambulance gurney. Voices were kept low as it was 11:30 pm and residents were sleeping. Both the nurse and I commented on his head. It was fixed, unmoving, even though the gurney ran over a few bumps. His mouth was open, and he was breathing through it. It gave us our first impression that he was near death. His room was the farthest from the nursing station. It was a quieter part of the building. During the day an East facing picture window allowed marginal sunlight to filter in. The thought of the gentleman spending his last days in the sunshine helped us emotionally.

As we transferred the resident's body from the gurney to his bed, I noticed he was fully dressed. He was wearing pants, a button-down shirt and socks. I expected him to be wearing open back clothing. He wasn't. It would mean that he would have to be manhandled to get him undressed and into a hospital nightgown.

Normal clothes for residents confined to a wheelchair are open at the back, secured by snaps. This type of clothing allows the Care Aide to dress the resident while he is in bed before lifting him into his chair. These clothes also avoid having to turn the resident several times as would happen if normal clothes were used, as was the case.

The nurse assisted me in rolling him to one side so I could pull down one sleeve of his shirt. It was then I noticed a dressing on his shoulder. It was drenched in a purulent discharge that had a foul smell.

We looked at one another. This wound should not have been there. There had been no indication of wounds on the nurse-to-nurse transfer documents. We rolled the resident to his other side to remove the opposite sleeve. There was a wound on his other shoulder. We also found a wound on his elbows. All the dressed wounds we could see were oozing a yellowish black discharge. The smell was deep, pungent. The smell of death. Slowly we continued.

Naked, the resident lay on top of the bed. He didn't shiver; at the end of life, we don't. As we undressed him, we did not fully comprehend the state of his body. We scoured every inch of him. In all, we found thirty-two 2nd and 3rd stage ulcers. Although all had had dressings applied, each was oozing. The ulcers on his coccyx were a rare 4th degree. They were so deep that we could easily see the fascia and in one small spot we were certain we could see the spine.

We also found significantly deep wounds on both hips, knees, ankles and one big toe. The wounds on our resident's hips had travelled deep into his legs making them difficult to clean and to apply treatment dressings. It was the worst case of skin destruction I have ever seen. It was the worst smell I have ever encountered.

Bed sores or ulcers come in four distinct stages.

Stage I

The beginning stage of a pressure sore has the following characteristics:

- The skin is not broken.
- The skin appears red on people with lighter skin colour, and the skin doesn't briefly lighten (blanch) when touched.
- On people with darker skin, the skin may show discoloration, and it doesn't blanch when touched.
- The site may be tender, painful, firm, soft, warm or cool compared with the surrounding tissue

Stage II

- The outer layer of skin and part of the underlying layer of skin is damaged or lost.
- The wound may be shallow and pinkish or red.

- The wound may look like a fluid-filled blister or a ruptured blister.

Stage III

the ulcer is a deep wound:
- The loss of skin usually exposes some fat.
- The ulcer looks crater-like.
- The bottom of the wound may have some yellowish dead tissue.
- The damage may extend beyond the primary wound below layers of healthy skin.

Stage IV

The ulcer shows large-scale loss of tissue:
- The wound may expose muscle, bone or tendons.
- The bottom of the wound likely contains dead tissue that's yellowish or dark and crusty.
- The damage often extends beyond the primary wound below layers of healthy skin.
- Unstageable(sic)
- A pressure ulcer is considered unstageable(sic) if its surface is covered with yellow, brown, black or dead tissue. It's not possible to see how deep the wound is.

Common sites of pressure sores

For people who use a wheelchair, pressure sores often occur on skin over the following sites:
- Tailbone or buttocks
- Shoulder blades and spine
- Backs of arms and legs where they rest against the chair

For people who are confined to bed, common sites include the following:
- Back or sides of the head
- Rim of the ears
- Shoulders or shoulder blades

- Hip, lower back or tailbone
- Heels, ankles and skin behind the knees (Mayo Clinic)

Understanding that the resident may have been able to feel pain, we gingerly removed each dressing to expose the wounds. As we did so the air became thick with the stench of death. We countered by breathing through our mouths.

We couldn't help but wonder how our resident arrived in such a degrading state. In health care, a multi-disciplinary team is usually established to approach the situation with a feasible care plan. The team members should include:

- A primary care physician who oversees the treatment plan
- A physician or nurse specialising in wound care
- Nurses or medical assistants who provide both care and education for managing wounds
- A physical therapist who helps with improving mobility
- A dietician who monitors nutritional needs and recommends an appropriate diet
- Care Aides who will carry out part of the treatment plan.

The basic care for a resident with ulcers is not difficult, but it does take teamwork and dedication. The care for our resident should have included:

Repositioning.

This resident should have been repositioned at least every two hours.
 Special turning sheets are used to assist caregivers. These sheets allow for easier turning and reduce friction and skin tears.
Cleansing of faecal material from the residents perineum and ensuring it dry before applying a clean pad.

Using support surfaces.

Special mattresses were available at the time. They would help relieve pressure over bony prominences.
Cleaning and dressing wounds

Care that helps with healing of the wound includes the following:

Cleaning. It's essential to keep wounds clean to prevent infection. If the affected skin is not broken (a stage I wound), a gentle wash with water and mild soap and pat dry Is all that is needed. An open sore (stage II, III, IV) on the other hand, is always treated by a nurse. She should use saltwater (saline) solution to cleanse the wound each time the dressing is changed.

Applying dressings. A dressing promotes healing by keeping a wound moist, creating a barrier against infection and keeping the surrounding skin dry. Dressing choices include films, gauzes, gels, foams and treated coverings. A combination of dressings may be used.

The doctor or wound nurse specialist selects a dressing based on a number of factors. These include the size and severity of the wound, the amount of discharge, and the ease of placing and removing the dressing. (National pressure ulcer advisory panel)

 The nurse asked me to phone the Director of Care and inform her of the situation. I left the nurse who had already begun to remove the contaminated dressings. I told the DOC that nothing was mentioned on the transfer papers about the resident's skin condition. After explaining what was found and the number of wounds associated with the emaciated body, I was told to photograph everything, the resident himself and every wound and location. There was an obvious need to collect evidence. I later found out the photographs were taken to avoid any risk of litigation by the resident's family.

 In all, I took forty-eight photographs. I then began to assist the nurse in dressing every wound. Each wound had to be cleansed with saline to remove surface debris. The wounds were then dressed. The wound on the coccyx was rather difficult and needed to be packed with sponges before finally being dressed. The most difficult of them all were the two wounds on each hip. They had burrowed deep under the skin. One had burrowed four inches.

The nurse slowly removed the packing. It was a long, half-inch wide, snake-like dressing. It oozed black skin and pus. There are no words to describe the smell. The resident was unconscious and almost certainly in a coma. As usual, we followed the strictest rule of conduct. And as we were both horrified at what we saw, we said nothing. We continued with our work in virtual silence.

It took three hours to complete the task, a task that would have to be repeated every day. After finishing, we searched for a pan for charcoal briquettes. We hoped it would help absorb some of the odour. It didn't work.

The resident passed away two weeks later. I never knew if he suffered through this abhorrent attack on his body. There is no doubt in my mind his prior treatments, if any, did not work. His care team should have had a different approach. His transfer papers did not tell the whole truth. This was, I believe, a wanton case of abuse.

I have known better times with residents with deep stage IV ulcers. In one instance we managed to repair that wound and return her skin to health.

She arrived at the facility where I worked with a large, deep ulcer on her coccyx. It measured ten centimetres in diameter. It was deep enough that I could have put my entire fist into the wound. As with the previous resident's wounds, this one smelled truly awful.

She was in a state of unconsciousness for two weeks. During that time, we set to work. Dressings were changed as per protocol. She was turned every two hours and was never left on her back. When she did awaken, she was fed high protein foods.

When she was finally conscious, she told me that all she wanted to do was die. She said that she did she not want to be in the nursing home, and she was more than embarrassed at her body smelling so vile. I told her that given time; she would be fine. We would fix her wound. She would find friends in the home.

Every night I worked she would say the same thing. She just wanted to die. I would always retort that I would not let her die, not until she was healthy. Then, I told her, she could do whatever she wanted.

Our treatments continued unabated for six months. Our resident was turned in bed every two hours. When in her wheelchair, she was shifted every hour. Eventually, she regained sufficient upper body strength to perform that task herself. Her dressings were changed as per dressing protocol.

After six months, the wound had healed. Fresh pink skin had grown over the large fissure. Although there was a large dip over her coccyx, the ulcer had completely disappeared. It was a triumph for tenacity and the correct team response to a crisis.

However, this treatment was not the case in every Long-Term Care facility. In one facility, they failed to reposition high-risk demented residents for at least six hours. I charged this facility with abuse.

THE CATYLIST

I contacted Cam Broten on March 24, 2015, regarding an article in the Saskatoon Star Phoenix. Mr Broten had raised concern about the staffing levels in a nursing home in Swift Current, Saskatchewan. He stated that the home had a staffing level of one staff to twelve residents and he thought that was outrageous. I mentioned this not only to the oncoming day crew but the following night shift as well.

The following evening, I mentioned the article to my partner and the RN. I laughed, saying: "I wish we had the same ratios." It took me two weeks of careful thought before I once again raised the issue. That shift was quiet. The residents were having a good quality sleep, something I strived for, for without that sleep dementia residents tend to be more anxious and aggressive during the day.

The spare time allowed me to draft the following email to Mr Broten. It was truthful. Yet, no one has come forward to refute my assertions.

I work at a Long Term Care facility in Saskatoon working nights. As with many other facilities, we work with less than a minimal amount of staff. Indeed, on several occasions, night staff have been told by management that we do work short. However, we have as yet to see any movement from management to correct the situation. It is our fervent belief staffing levels for nights are reduced in order to facilitate a better bottom line. The statistics for night shift staffing levels that follow have remained consistent for the previous 4 years. The numbers shown are correct at the time and date of this email and are as follows. Staff (Continuing Care Aide) to residents 1:23. If we remove hours taken for meal/coffee breaks, then the ratio rises to 1:28. In the secure (dementia) unit we have a ratio of 1:18 with one staff member being on their own for up to 3 hours per shift. I work in the secure unit. We have 32 residents with all in early to late 3rd stage dementia. The residents are very difficult to work with, with many wandering, some relieving themselves on the floor with others bed ridden and always 1 or 2 facing death. There are up to 10 people that need to have their night pads changed, and many of them need to be turned to help alleviate the risk of bed sores developing. Unfortunately, these residents cannot receive the care they need until 0400 (4 AM) due to staffing levels. Many are so wet we have to change all their bedding. And all will have been sleeping in one position for 6 - 12 hours depending on when they were assisted to bed. This, I firmly believe, is an absolute abuse of the resident. I am, of course, implicit in this abuse only by virtue of instructions from the duty RN. Further to this abuse, staff members have been abused by residents by way of being punched, kicked, or pinched especially when the Care Aide is required to work with residents without the use of any available assistance. There are a plethora of abuse stories I could share. However, there would be insufficient space in this email. I, therefore, am attempting to document every incident of resident abuse I have personally witnessed. So far I have approximately 23 serious incidents and counting. For your efforts in trying to bring the government to heel on health care issues, I thank you.

At that point, I had no inkling that I would become, what I now believe, the infamous whistleblower.

In my email, I mentioned that I had twenty-three examples of abuse. These examples have been collected during my past eleven years as a CCA. In a subsequent email to Mr Broten, I informed him that I had been writing a manuscript of resident abuse that I had personally witnessed. I explained that in every case complete confidentiality had been maintained.

The untitled manuscript had been underway for seven years. It would take the ensuing charges of resident abuse and the unfolding political nonsense to bring it to fruition.

I then started to offer the investigator my opinion of why abuse was occurring. Approximately once every six weeks, night shift had a meeting with management. It was designed to flush out any problems that might be occurring. It was also designed to heighten our spirits and to give us a verbal slap on the back with a, you're doing a wonderful job, well done.' I always followed the reassurance with, 'don't throw accolades, throw cash.' In those days' witticism helped carry the night.

It was at these meetings that the difficulties with getting residents dressed for the day surfaced. I pointed out that many were still sleeping and that I was reluctant to wake them. We were told, and in no uncertain terms, residents in dementia were to sleep until they woke. This was a directive from management. Not only was it taken to heart, but became part of our morning routine.

Although my charge of abuse was against residents, staff were also abused. One incident still horrifies me.

One morning all residents were sleeping. My partner and I searched for something to do if only to keep us awake. Suppositories were supposed to be given in the morning by the day crew. They were in the best position to give the proper toileting care. Both my partner and I decided to assist the day crew by giving the suppositories. The day crew thanked us profusely. Although a minor benefit to them, it did relieve them of an extra burden placed on their shift.

Everything went well until one morning several residents were awake and needed to get dressed. Our instructions were clear. If a resident was awake, he/she needed to get dressed and taken to the dining room. The resident could be observed more closely in the confines of that room. Anything else was secondary. Safety and security of the resident were paramount.

That morning we did not deliver the suppositories. The duty day nurse (always an LPN in dementia) became very belligerent when asking why we had not given the suppositories. I explained the rationale and the fact that we were following protocol. She became very angry with me as I explained that we only started to give out the suppositories because there was no work to do. I further stated that at first, it was a voluntary act, to help the day crew. I continued with: "You then expected it of us, and now you demand that we give out the suppositories. We are not going to do all your bloody work!"

I took the helm of the argument and went head to head with my superior. It was something that should not have happened. The night RN should have carried the banner of diktat informing the LPN of the established protocols. She didn't. She begged off. She did not have the whither all to stand up to a much stronger person. That morning a plan was set in motion that would be the most disgusting act any nurse could perpetrate.

A few mornings later a night crew made up of a part-time and a casual CCA had finished their work. No one was awake. The suppositories had been laid out on the report room desk. I had previously come to an agreement with the LPN that, should time permit, we would give the suppositories. This morning, however, the two CCA's had decided to watch television in the resident lounge instead of doing their assigned work. A day shift CCA saw them and raised the proverbial roof. All the day crew were upset, and they remained so up until the evening crew came on board.

In their anger or disgust (I was never to find out), the day crew had purposely not delivered the suppositories, leaving that chore for the evening shift. The LPN (now working her scheduled evening shift) brought her plan to fruition. It was time to get back at the night crew who had refused to give out the suppositories and to deliver a message to me personally. She instructed her Care Aides to give the suppositories at 10:30 pm. It was a stupid thing to do. It was an ignorant act. It was a failure of everything she had been taught in training. She had failed the trust of the residents, her staff, and her profession.

As I started the shift, I was informed of the very late delivery of the suppositories. I was annoyed but took the news in a high spirit refusing to be drawn into a fight. At midnight, the RN arrived for shift report. It was then that she discovered what had happened. She also was annoyed. However, the deed had been done. Justice, I assumed, must surely follow.

Before justice could follow, one of the residents was awake and walking the hallways. The suppository given her was working. She had filled her night pad to overflowing with her faeces. There was a trail of it on the floor. She had tried to remove her pad but was successful only in covering her hands with human defecation. My partner and I quickly got to work. We cleaned her up and got her back to bed. Within minutes, another of the three unfortunate residents was up and walking out of her room. Her pad was full of BM, but it managed to stay in her pad. The third resident would awaken within a short while.

The first resident up would repeat her behaviour several times that night, not settling until after 3:00 am. The other two would continue to stay awake most of the night. Each showed definitive signs of anxiousness and discomfort. There is no doubt each resident was psychologically damaged. It was not natural for them to soil themselves. They were on a toileting plan; had they received the suppositories in the morning, they would have had, as was usual, a comfortable, restful night.

I was responsible for all thirty-two residents from 1:30 am until my partner returned from her work on another floor. During that time, I looked after not only those three unfortunate ladies that had soiled themselves, but I was also responsible for doing a breathing round and putting other residents to bed. It was a tremendous amount of work saturated by the stupidity of the LPN.

I have many friends within the nursing community. To each, they believe the LPN was vindictive and spiteful. She used her office to 'get back at me.' She should have been held accountable for her actions. Many of my colleagues stated that the abuse was sufficient to warrant severe discipline. All believed termination to be appropriate discipline. To my knowledge, the night RN failed to report the incident to management. As far as I am aware, nothing untoward happened to the LPN. Staff relations hit a new low that night. It was never to recover.

The same day I received this email:

As I drill deeper into the alleged resident abuse, I will need to email you a few more times for further clarification. My apologies in advance. These are complicated and serious issues requiring attention to detail.

It appeared to me as though my charges of abuse were being taken seriously. I did not know, however, how twisted and sordid the entire process would become.

On May 08, 2015, I received the following email:

Hi there I need to discuss the resident abuse allegations in person.

The investigator had determined that the allegations were too serious to deal with over email. He added that we would not be dealing with accusations made against me by my co-workers at that time but with my allegations of abuse against residents. He then added that he thought the meeting would last about two hours.

THE DRINKER

Several years ago, Long-Term Care Facilities underwent major changes in their approach to care. Originally, care plans for residents lay within the institutional model, a model based on the needs of staff. It was a model of which Florence Nightingale herself would have approved. A military type work environment where everyone knew their place, meals were served at a certain time, residents were woken at 6:00 am and put to bed by 10:00 pm. Staff were in control and authoritarianism ruled the roost.

Times had changed. A new wave of non-conformists had rolled in. Their teachings seemed to make sense. Gone was the militarism of the past. In came the psychological approach to Long Term Care. Residents embraced the new ideas. Management saw a different breed of client, happier, more willing to do things, to become more independent and to live the life they wanted, not what staff wanted.

The new model turned everything 180 degrees. Care had become resident-centred. The resident now dictated to his/her care staff when they would get up when they would eat when they would use the bathroom. Most importantly they dictated when they would go to bed.

Many of the old guard disliked the new model. Some abhorred it; others vowed not to work under the new conditions. And a few walked away from a lifelong career. Care Aides had to change the way they looked at the needs of residents. Although they still worked as a team, moving sequentially from door to door, getting residents up for the day was now a thing of the past. It would become haphazard. The first awake, regardless of where they were along the corridor, became the first to be helped to get dressed. Running up and down the hallway took extra time. It made extra work.

Staff were angry. Productivity dropped. A non-caring attitude began to raise its ugly head, and with the ability to settle the issue, management refused to spend any money to make amends. Management was aware there would be no new staff hired to compensate for the extra work. After all, there was still the same number of residents. And by playing with numbers, management's favourite pastime, the ratio of Care Aides to residents remained the same.

For those Care Aides that hung on, it took time for them to settle into a non-routine environment. However, dietary and housekeeping remained upset. No one quite knew how many residents were going to show for meals. And housekeeping didn't know when rooms would be empty.

A more difficult situation arose at meal times. The dining room had enough seating for half the residents. It became more than annoying when some residents wanted to change their sitting times. I heard the term "a fucking mess" many times as Care Aides and Dietary fought to bring the situation under control. In the time I was there, control would be the last word I would use. It almost turned to mass hysteria.

One resident took full advantage of the new model. As adults, residents should have been allowed to consume alcohol at any time. Before the new rules came into effect, alcohol was stored in the medication room under lock and key. It was controlled and distributed by the nurse (many times punishment was meted out by way of refusal to hand out alcohol). But the new rules allowed for residents to store their liquor in their rooms. Nurses were upset.

A major part of their punishment strategy had been taken away from them. Their workload increased as did their responsibilities. It was also becoming more difficult to keep track of their staff. It was as if the word 'care' had flitted out of the window to be replaced with apprehensiveness.

Care was now controlled by the resident, and an air of discomfort settled over the staff. In the new model, the resident could also drink outside as long as he remained on the property. In this case, the resident was cognizant and fully aware of what he was doing. The result of this new model would turn out to be extremely dangerous. It would almost kill him.

He was young to be in a Long-Term Care Facility, far too young. In his mid-fifties, he felt out of place with residents whose age averaged well over eighty years. He looked old, bedraggled with deep scarring lines etched in his gaunt, colourless face. A smile across his thin lips was something I never saw. Sitting alone in his wheelchair, I never saw him speak to anyone. He was a loner; someone wrapped up in a life of cruelty.

One evening he started a conversation with me. We were out on the porch, he in his wheelchair and me on a bench. He wanted to talk, to get something off his chest. I was the only male Care Aide. I automatically became his target. Far from being bothered by his intrusion, I enjoyed our conversation.

He told me that he had worked hard as a truck driver, moving old asbestos from work sites to a garbage dump. At the time, he didn't know the dangers of asbestos; very few did. He described how every day he was awash with extremely fine particles of the deadly material. He would often walk through clouds of fine dust to get to his truck cab. It was a good living, and he enjoyed his job.

It would be years before he began to have difficulty breathing. He was astonished when he first heard his diagnosis and decidedly scared when he heard his prognosis; there was no chance to fight the disease. The doctor told him that he had asbestosis. Death was inevitable. And at the stage he was at it would be sooner rather than later. He had been told that asbestosis was linked to chrysotile fibres. Chrysotile is one of the six known types of asbestos. Exposure occurs when someone breathes in the dangerous fibres. Extended exposure can lead to an accumulation of the fibres in lung tissues, setting the stage for long-term fibrosis (scarring). Over time, lung tissues thicken, causing pain and restricting breathing. (healthline).

He had all the symptoms expected with the disease: a persistent cough that produced mucus, chest tightness, chest pain, loss of appetite and a crackling sound in his lungs while inhaling. He was aware that the condition was becoming worse.

I was a new Care Aide. I did what I was told. This resident, however, was to teach me the true art of care: talking to residents; understanding them and giving empathy where and when it was needed. And yet I was also to learn that many in my profession did not measure up to what would become my personal standards, standards that had been drilled into me in college. At this point, all I knew was that the young trucker was often in a wheelchair. The simple exertion to move brought on rapid, shallow and painful breathing.

One sultry evening our trucker had spent several hours outside, under the covered porch drinking beer. The beer was cheap. It came in a plastic two-litre bottle. But it was over six percent alcohol, and he seemed to revel in losing himself in the suds. It was companionship. In the nursing home, he was alone, hermit-like and antisocial and that's the way he liked it.

The nursing home was attached to a church. Most of the residents admitted were of this denomination. Deeply rooted, they formed a bond that carried them into the netherworld. A good number of the older staff also belonged to this doctrine. Without question, drinking and smoking were frowned upon. It was no wonder those that belonged to this religion disliked him.

Matters were made worse when it was discovered that he was an atheist. A Care Aide was looking through his chart one day when she came across his nurse-to-nurse transfer documents. Under religion, the damning name had been written. As Care Aides, we are supposed to treat all residents the same, irrespective of their religious beliefs. This, surprisingly, was not done. He was singled out. It almost cost him his life.

That fateful evening, I found the resident outside. He was in his wheelchair. Two empty bottles of beer were on his lap. I noticed that he was having difficulty breathing. His respiration was fast and shallow. His fingers had turned blue (cyanosis). It is a condition indicative of low oxygen in the blood. He was in serious trouble. His body needed oxygen and quickly. As an Emergency Medical Technician (EMT), I fully understood what was happening.

Respiratory shock occurs when there is insufficient oxygen in the body. The heart and brain, major recipients of oxygen, fail to function properly. Thus, blood flow is reduced. This results in cellular destruction. Cellular destruction of the heart creates a situation where the heart works so inefficiently, cardiac arrest is a definite possibility. (/www.nhlbi.nih.gov/health/health)

As I took him back to his room, we passed the nursing station. The duty nurse was talking on the telephone (later, I was told that it was to a friend). I informed her that the resident was having great difficulty breathing. Believing the nurse would take responsibility for the resident, I left him in his room and went about my work assisting others to bed.

Nearly an hour had passed before I returned to the resident's room. I wanted to see how he was responding to treatment. When I arrived, I found him slumped over, breathing very rapidly. His respirations were very shallow and rapid. He was sweating profusely. I could hear with ease the crackling sounds from his lungs. He had gone into respiratory shock. He was dying.

I immediately called the nurse. She was still talking on the phone. She appeared unconcerned. She looked over at me. With a flippant look, she returned to her telephone conversation. I had the impression the phone call was more important.

I shouted at her, "NURSE! STAT!"

It had the desired effect. Putting the phone down, the RN rushed to the resident's room. When she arrived, he was in full respiratory shock. His hands and feet were cyanotic, and there were signs of mottling (a condition where the blood pressure is so low that blood does not reach the extremities. It's usually seen within twenty-four hours of death). It appeared as though the nurse herself had gone into shock.

She stood at the door and stammered, "What should I do?"

At first, I was taken aback. A Registered Nurse not knowing what to do? It was the most basic of human function, breathing oxygen. How could she not know that? It took several seconds before I responded.

"He needs oxygen," I answered loudly and with frustration in my voice. I was trying to remove his sweat filled jacket as I told her to "get the concentrator and nasal prongs, and hurry." I then added, "Get someone to phone 911."

A concentrator is a machine that draws oxygen from the air. Oxygen is delivered to the resident by way of two small tubes that rest on the underside of the resident's nose. As she arrived with the machine, I was the one who had to plug it in to get it working. When done, I set about placing the nasal prongs on the resident. The nurse just stood in the doorway not moving. It was an emergency, and she was doing nothing to help. She stood there, a brick out of a wall, useless. I didn't have time to be annoyed. That would come later.

Due to the resident's medical condition, I could only deliver two percent oxygen. It was sufficient to keep him oxygenated until the ambulance arrived. Barely a word was spoken to the resident, all my thoughts ripping through college books read long ago on oxygenation and respiratory shock.

When the ambulance crew arrived, they asked several questions of myself and the nurse. They had discovered that he had not received any medication. They quickly put him on medication that was delivered through a mask directly to his lungs. Within minutes the resident began to 'pink up'. His skin began to turn a normal colour. Breathing became noticeably easier, and his sweating eased. He was not out of danger, but he had started on the road to recovery.

The nurse had vanished. She had returned to the nursing station preparing the paperwork that would be needed by the receiving hospital.

As I watched the ambulance pull away, I had little time to think of what had transpired. I still had several residents to assist to bed. And although other staff had finished putting their residents to bed, none would help me. It felt strange. I had believed resident care was a priority and that teamwork was essential in Long Term Care.

Teamwork in long-term care is often a misnomer. Care Aides are responsible for their residents and will not automatically assist a colleague in need of help. On far too many occasions residents would have to wait for their Care Aide to put them to bed even though other Aides were sitting resting. Although I have known many excellent Care Aides, who would help a colleague in need, in this case, I was on my own. This strange practice appears to be systemic and creates tension among many care workers and residents alike.

The next morning, when my brain had settled, I gave deep thought to the previous evening's emergency. In point form, I had written notes on the embarrassing situation. Included were the 5 W's: when, where, why, who and what. I had also included key times of certain incidents.

I felt the situation needed to be reported. I sent a memo to the Director of Care. Certainly, the nurse's skills were poor. I was convinced had she been there on her own the resident would have died. That, to me, was totally unacceptable.

Work-related incidents concerning nurses are generally reported by Care Aides or other staff, housekeeping, dietary, etc. Rarely do nurses make mistakes. But when they do honesty usually comes to the fore. For instance, if a drug error is made the nurse is required to fill out paperwork explaining the situation. The resident's doctor is apprised of the situation as well as the DOC. We are all human; nurses are no exception, and when we make a mistake, especially in health care, we own up to it.

A few days later I was called into the Director of Care's office. My report was on her desk. I gave a verbal explanation regarding the incident. She was aware of my Emergency Medical Technician credentials. Thus, the meeting was cordial but exhaustive. I was there to explain what had happened, why I believed the resident was in danger. Why I thought the nurse failed in her duty.

Approximately three weeks later I was summoned to a meeting at what was now my previous workplace (I had accepted a new position at another facility). When I arrived, there were several people in the room. One was from the nurse's union, others from the Health Region. The Director of Care was also present. There was one more person in the room, but I was not aware of who they were. I was pummelled with questions for twenty to thirty minutes regarding the incident. I answered all of their questions as truthfully as I could.

When asked my opinion of the event I clearly stated that I believed the nurse was incompetent. That the resident would have died had I, or another Care Aide, not been present.

I found it brutal to report another staff member on their lack of skills. The thought of doing so still haunts me. However, it did pave the way for my understanding of how nurses and management protect one another, for the nurse was neither asked to resign nor was she fired.

I'm never one to see punishment handed down for an error, a mistake, especially if no one is injured. I am one that believes people must learn from their mistakes.

I sometimes wonder; did I make a mistake? Was I too aggressive, was she scared of my approach? Should I have stood back and let her take control of the situation? And then I remember the resident's face. Ashen grey, it was pleading, crying, dying. I could do nothing but take immediate action.

No, I don't regret what I did.

But it still bothers me.

SLAM DUNK

The two-hour meeting would stretch into an exhausting four-hour interrogation. It would be the start of my demise. If the investigation was a ship, then the investigator was the Captain. He made certain that should the ship sink it would be me who would go down with her. All had damned me.

I had no arguments with April 24, 2015, transcript of the first meeting with the investigator. I read every page and guarded each word jealousy. There were no damning statements in the document just clear and concise rules of play. I was to learn much later that my rep had difficulty with the transcript. She believed parts of the conversation were missing. She was a voracious taker of notes. During the investigation, I'm sure she must have filled two or three notebooks. Therefore, I took her analysis to heart. She would make her annoyance with the investigator's ideal of 'verbatim' felt at the meeting

My rationale for the abuse allegations had always been staff shortage. And although I answered all the investigator's questions in our correspondence, I didn't see any logic in me being involved in this part of the investigation. All he had to show was that under-staffing was the primary cause for delay in appropriate care for the residents. It wasn't rocket science, after all. Proof would be simple. Checking staff schedules would be sufficient to identify those shifts when we were short staffed. And he would only have to check the Care Aide's routine to confirm that he/she was left alone in dementia for up to four hours a night. It was, so I thought that simple. It should have been a slam-dunk!As we sat there, I sensed something was wrong. The same rat I smelled before came storming back, but this time it was a far stronger smell. Until the bitter end, I could never get rid of that smell. I wasn't stupid. I knew my reputation as a Care Aide was going to be thoroughly tested. My memory would be held up to ridicule. My job with the Saskatoon Health Region was on the line. Once more I had the distinct feeling I was going to fall, and hard.

As I sat in my employer's basement, in the old training room, I was happy to be with my union rep. She was armed with pen and notebook and ready for action. The investigator did what would become his usual routine by arriving in the room after everybody else. I was relieved the show was finally on the road. We were told that not only was he investigating the myriad of allegations against me, but he had been charged with investigating the abuse allegations as well.

In SHRA, Long Term Care resident's charting was done by exception. Or to put it another way only relevant information would be charted.

If a resident had two repeated incidents in two successive days that would signal the end of the charting for that incident. It would then become the resident's normal routine. If the routine changed, then it would be charted as an exception. And so it went. I was to learn that not charting every single incident would lead me to a fight for survival.

At eight in the morning, in my employer's basement training room, the second of four meetings began. I was asked to sit near the front of the room. Whatever was said would be recorded. Beside me, but a chair away was my union rep. To the left was a long desk that ran at a ninety-degree angle to my table. This was the investigator's throne, his command post. A laptop computer was in front of him.

On the table, opposite mine were several stacks of blue and white documents each neatly held together with elastic bands. These belonged to those deceased. They consisted of charts, nursing notes and other paraphernalia. The far desk, and opposite the investigator sat a young woman whose open laptop obscured her face. I was told that she was a transcriptionist and would type word for word all conversations.

This, we would later discover, was not quite the truth. Not every word was transcribed, and those that were faced some very sketchy editing.

With preliminaries out of the way, the questions started and they came thick and fast. It wouldn't take long before I considered myself being on trial and not the system. The Care Aides I had worked with had not come forward in my support even though they had witnessed everything I had and had supported my position. Had they done so I would have felt more comfortable. But they didn't. They took the opposite view. They were prepared to lie and face the distinct possibility of perjury should I have decided to litigate.

Without the strength of truth from my co-workers, I would have to advocate for the residents on my own.

"What had I seen on this resident that led me to believe she had been abused?" And so the inquisition began.

I told the investigator both hips had what I considered stage one ulcers. Her ears had pressure marks as did the sides of both feet. I compared the marks with medical photographs and definitions of ulcers. The pictures and definitions showed ulcers ranging from stage one through stage four. I was, without any shadow of a doubt, looking at stage-one ulceration.

I was asked for my title and job description. After informing the investigator what he already knew, I was told me that I did not have the authority to give an assessment of wounds on a resident.

"Why then," I asked, "is there a diagnostic chart in the nursing supply room? That chart," I continued, "gives clear photographs and identification details of ulcers. The chart clearly identifies skin ulcers from stage one to stage four. With this chart, I identified the ulcers on the resident to be stage one. If she were to be turned every four hours, as I was doing until taking ill in December of 2014, then these ulcers would all but disappear."

He then informed me that the resident's physician had looked at her and the areas in question and had concluded that she did not have ulcers.

"That", I said, "did not surprise me. If the resident had turned every four hours, as was the practice before Christmas of 2014, then there wouldn't be any ulcers. First stage ulcers are the easiest to treat. Keep the resident off the area and voila, cured."

In nursing, there is indisputable proof that physicians are treated like Gods. It appeared as though this was the case with this resident. The investigator had asked the physician whether he believed his patient had been abused and whether she had ulceration of her hips and other identified parts of her body.

The resident's physician replied by letter. He found no incidents of either abuse or skin damage. I was not privy to the document and had to take the investigator at his word. I questioned whether the physician performed a full assessment. I explained that the resident is usually one of the first to be readied for the day. As she is non-ambulatory, she is placed in her wheelchair with a tray in front of her. I then went on the attack.

"The doctor would almost certainly arrive after she was in her wheelchair," I said, thinking hard about my next sentence. "Due to the location of the injuries, a complete assessment would have to be performed with her laying down. It certainly could not be performed in her chair. There is no doubt she would have to be placed on her bed. That would require a mechanical lift. A mechanical lift cannot be used unless there are two trained people to operate it. Either the LPN and a Care Aide or two Care Aides would have to perform the procedure.

"Once on her bed the resident's clothing would have to be removed to examine the resident's hips. There is no doubt the physician would not perform this procedure if there were Care Aides present." He tried to stop me, but I would have none of it. I needed to ask one question after my dissertation. The investigator knew where I was going. He understood all too well that I was placing him in a trap. I sensed he was preparing his rebuttal. I continued.

"So, if the doctor did show up to examine the resident, and if he did do a thorough examination as he suggests in his report to you, then there must be at least two Care Aides who witnessed his actions. I'm curious, did you happen to interview those two Care Aides?"

I had stepped over the bounds of decency. In health care doctors are Gods. They are the means to climb the ladder of success. The allegations of abuse had received province-wide media attention. I had been interviewed several times on television news programs. From Vancouver to Toronto, newspapers across the country had picked up the news feed. This investigator, I believe, saw a means to an end. If he could prove that abuse did not happen, then he would be looking to climb a few steps of his own.

I then decided to turn the proverbial thumbscrews just a little more. I forcibly told him had the doctor been there at 4:00 am then he would have seen the tell-tale marks of ulcerating skin. I then asked if he knew any doctor that would attend a resident at that time in the morning. He didn't answer.

The investigator was visibly upset. He snapped back: "Are you suggesting the doctor is lying?"

"That is for you to determine," I said, somewhat wryly. "What I'm suggesting is that you should interview others who were witness to his examination, just to make sure." I wanted to say, "to satisfy that eager investigative mind of yours," but I held that in check. I had already proven a point, and it felt good.

Of course, I didn't want him to consider for a moment that I believed anything any doctor said without the rigours of cross-examination. And cross-examination was one luxury I did not and would not have.

The minor scuffle was over. It was short, a quick jab, just enough to keep the investigator alert. He quickly realised that I was not the sort of person to lay down and plead for mercy. These little jabs would be more frequent as time went on. And with each one he bled just a little. The sword in my heart, however, was going in ever deeper.

We got back to the subject at hand. "Did you consult anyone with your concerns about the resident's health?"

"But of course," I said, looking at my interrogator. "I informed the duty nurse of my concerns. I told her that according to the routine I was not allowed to turn the resident until four in the morning. I told her that that was a full six hours after the previous shift had ended. I also told her that there would be other residents in the same position unless we did something, and quickly. I then said that I thought the problem stemmed from a lack of staff. "We just don't have adequate personnel to perform the proper standard of care expected of us, me. We do not have the ability to manage our time effectively." I then added: "Had I expected any sign of conventional wisdom, I certainly did not get it from the RN."

She told me that, with one exception, there were no residents that needed turning at night. She identified the resident and said that she had Multiple Sclerosis and was unable to move any part of her body without assistance. She went on to say that the resident was cognitive. She would become uncomfortable, especially if she were left in one position for an extended period. She rattled on, seemingly annoyed. Her diatribe was becoming sillier and, to me, more peculiar especially as it was coming from a Registered Nurse. She finished by saying that that was the reason our Multiple Sclerosis resident was the only one of one hundred and thirty-eight others in the facility who needed turning.

"Then what happened?" The nurse left the unit obviously aware that I was annoyed, angry. I do not remember whether there was a witness in the room. All I remember was the terrible, unprofessional treatment afforded my residents and me.

The next shift the nurse tried to appease me by calmly reiterating what she had said the previous night. Her voice was softer, almost apologetic. However, the message was the same, and no amount of arguing would shake her resolve. There was to be no resolution. It quickly dissolved into her way or the highway. Personally, I thought the highway appeared to be the better route.

I surmised that if I could not do my job effectively, which was to advocate competently for the residents in my charge, then there seemed little point in staying. Something deep inside me screamed out, 'abandon ship'. Within an hour, I was searching the SHRA website for work.

"If you thought that abuse was happening and your supervisor was taking no action, then why did you not report it to management?"

It was a reasonable question, a question that had a definitive answer. I told the investigator that night staff have a meeting with management approximately every six weeks. At least one of the managers was always present. Care Aides reported any problems and concerns that we faced during our shifts. The problems with dementia were always reported to the RN first. That followed proper protocol. If she failed in her response, then it would be raised at the meeting.

We always hoped to get a more positive hearing from management over issues that concerned us. How misguided we were. Had I suspected for a moment that we would be getting little more than a passive hearing then I certainly would not have wasted my time and effort.

I should have known that my concern in dementia would be muted. I always believed that a proper standard of care expected by residents and their families would overshadow management's need for budgetary restraint. And no matter how many issues were raised, the answer was always the same. "We do not have sufficient funding for extra staff."

A case in point was the issue of malfunctioning radios. These walkie-talkies were essential for the smooth operation of the nursing home at night. With only one Care Aide on dementia for up to four hours, effective communication was vital.

As the new building opened, cheap Motorola radios were used to communicate between staff. They were rarely successful. Each had a habit of failing after a few months. The interference was startling. It was not possible to communicate with anyone, even on the same floor let alone in the same building. But those cheap little radios were our only contact with the nurse. They were vital tools. They were there to protect both residents and staff. They became a very frustrating tool. Occasionally they would work. Often, we just left them in the charger. Over the years, three new radio sets were purchased. As usual, within three months they failed. I have little knowledge of radios. But I do have a lot of common sense. I discovered a possible reason for it. And I developed what I thought was a sensible and viable solution.

During one night shift, a resident had punched a hole in a wall. Through the hole, I saw a metal stud. I quickly understood that we were in a spider web of metal. I believed that the metallic spider web scrambled the weak radio waves. In my youth, I listened to short wave radio. I was aware of things that blocked or reduced the radio's broadcast strength. I assumed that this alone would cause significant interference. I then considered the radios themselves.

Advertised as having a broadcast range of twenty to twenty-eight kilometres, they, in fact, had a broadcast range of fewer than 400 metres, and that was on a good day. I read the fine print. Atmospheric and ground interference would greatly reduce their range. I then considered the federal broadcast legislation concerning these radios. Suffice it to say; they were not destined to work well.

These radios were used to contact the nurse. They were there to ensure the safety of staff and resident at night. That communication line failed. For four years' management did nothing. For those four years, they had little regard for the safety and security of both residents and staff. It was abysmal.

At our meetings, I told management the only answer to the radio problem was to rent high powered devices. I had used this type of radio in my past working life. They were reliable and worked extremely well in all environments. I had raised this resolution each time the use of malfunctioned radios was mentioned. But as usual the damning answer -- "We can't afford it" -- raised its ugly head.

The problem concerning the radios was made worse by the nurse agreeing with management. The radios weren't essential was the main thrust of her argument. We had lived without them for many a shift, and we managed. Therefore, we didn't need them. I wanted to counter with: if a car goes down a straight road, does it need a steering wheel? I thought better of it. I was already upset, and I didn't see the need to make matters worse.

I tried a different tack. I asked management what would happen if the night aide working on dementia was attacked by a resident. How could that Care Aide communicate with the nurse? The only way would be to get to the office phone. If the attack occurred at the farthest point in the building, it could cause very serious issues. Even though we recently had an incident where it took five staff to control a violent resident, my argument gained no ground. We could use call bells, came the reply.

Call bells were not used in dementia. However, each room was equipped with a call bell panel. This panel consisted of three distinct coloured buttons. There was a green nurse button, a red emergency button and a yellow cancel button. Should the emergency button be pressed, the alarm would register on everyone's pager in real time, no delays. It seemed a logical answer to the chronic problem. But then, as always, I began to think of those "what if's."

The idea was that the nurse receiving the alarm would respond as quickly as possible. I had some serious issues with what I began to believe was a silly plan. What would happen if the attack occurred in the hallway? The answer was the stupidest ever given. I was told that we did not have any violent residents on the unit, so that shouldn't be a problem. The concern was more for residents that had fallen. I then dropped a mini-bombshell. I told management that our nurses did not carry their pagers, they never had. They always complained that they were a nuisance, always going off at the wrong time when they were busy. Management must have taken heed for a short while later, all staff, nurses included, were to carry their alarm pagers. A small victory, perhaps. Night RN's and LPN's had to toe the line. They were no longer able to avoid the alarm system. And it drove them nuts.

However, we were back to square one. No money for better radios, nurses who refused to carry pagers, and we were dealing with a most bizarre and somewhat deranged management. The night crew were becoming very frustrated. Most knew that it would take one of us to get beaten by a resident before any change would come about. Until then, irrational management personnel would not, or perhaps did not, realise the importance of these communication tools.

In January of 2015 management changed their ways. Something must have triggered their conscious minds for when I returned to work later that month large, high-powered radios awaited me. I was elated. Now I could be in contact with anybody anywhere in the building. The signal was crystal clear. A sense of relief filled me. I still thought management was stupid, but at least my message got through. However, I had forgotten about the nurses and their pagers. Every alarm the staff received was also triggered on the nurse's pagers. And woe befell us if we did not answer them in a timely fashion.

"Room so and so is buzzing," or "so and so is out of bed," and so it went. Their voices seemed filled with joyous venom, payback for spilling the beans on them not carrying their pagers

I had achieved success with the radios. I had surmounted the impossible and made management understand the dire need for them. I couldn't help but wonder if my other complaints of residents in distress would sink into management's collective minds. I attempted to raise the issue of staff shortage and the effect on the standard of care expected. I was a little naïve for the subject once again fell on deaf ears. The damning part of it all was they voluntarily told us we were working short-staffed.

THE BM

When he arrived on the unit, we could still smell the fresh paint and touch unmarked walls. Many residents in dementia were called wanderers, those who had the ability to walk (ambulate). Although the unit took on the more degrading name, 'the lock up', its actual name was either the wandering unit or the secure unit. Inside the secure unit, all doors were lockable. Exiting dementia was by way of three electronic coded doors. It was a safe place for residents. Safety was the key word.

Residents with dementia and Alzheimer's disease have issues with their internal body clocks. They are often awake at night. Conversely, they tend to sleep during the day. It was not unusual to have up to eight residents walking about at night. And although they could do little harm to themselves, the potential to harm one another was high. Security, therefore, was a good part of my work. And that security was always put at risk when I was essentially abandoned, being arbitrarily mandated to work alone for up to four hours. And although those I worked with disputed this fact, the evidentiary proof was well established during the investigation.

During the first three years of the dementia unit being opened, my partner and I would have up to twelve residents dressed and ready for the day before our shift ended. It was a hectic time. An enjoyable time. It was the time when I learned more about the residents by observing the way they were; the way they walked, tried to talk and attempted to be a part of something, even though they didn't understand what that was. However, there was a sense of camaraderie, and when I sang well-known World War II songs, any number of them tried to join in.

More importantly, I learned their mood triggers, what angered them, what calmed them. It was information that stayed with me up to the end. It not only helped me communicate more effectively with them but gave me the confidence to help calm them when one of the triggers was accidentally squeezed.

My resident of whom I now speak was not considered a wanderer. He was, however, ambulatory. He would wake at night to toilet himself. He had the ability to put himself back to bed, and he did so without fuss. It made my life on the unit a little easier. He could be trusted to perform a normal human need, to relieve himself. He performed the task not only out of necessity but within the sphere of independence.

He was a good resident. He caused us little difficulty. When he awoke, we would assist him in getting ready for the day. He would select the clothes he wanted to wear, and with supervision, he could get dressed. He had the ability to button up his shirt (albeit with snap buttons). He could also secure his belt. His favourite task, however, was shaving. He would spend up to fifteen minutes buzzing his day-old stubble with his electric shaver.

When finished I would check his neck then tell him, "hey bud; you missed a bit." His smile was uplifting as he moved the razor to the rough spot. However, in dementia I knew all too well what I witnessed in those early days would not last. Indeed, it would be less than a year that I would have to help with his shaving. A few months later he had lost the ability to shave altogether.

He could still select the clothes that he wanted to wear, but he could no longer dress by himself. By this time the ability to toilet himself at night was over. One of the last vestiges of dignity had vanished into his tired, lost past. It was time for him to wear a full pad and allow Care Aides to change him at night. Dignity was gone. Independence exhausted. He now relied on around-the-clock care. If there are sad days in dementia, then these are they.

It wasn't long, perhaps three years from being admitted, but he became bed-ridden. He had both Alzheimer's and Parkinson's diseases. Residents with this disease, Lewy body, are particularly difficult to work with. Unfortunately, few of us working with this resident had any in-depth knowledge of it. And yet it is the second most diagnosed disease after Alzheimer's. However, few understood the disease more than I for I have a family member who is afflicted by it.

An overview of Lewy body dementia is perhaps warranted:

Lewy body dementia is a form of dementia that occurs because of abnormal deposits of a protein called alpha-synuclein inside the brain's nerve cells. These deposits are called "Lewy bodies," after the scientist who first described them. The deposits interrupt the brain's messages. Lewy body dementia usually affects the areas of the brain that involve thinking and movement. Why or how Lewy bodies form is unknown.

Lewy body dementia can occur by itself, or together with Alzheimer's disease or Parkinson's. (Alzheimer Society of Canada) The most common symptoms of LBD include Impaired thinking, such as loss of executive function (planning, processing information), memory, or the ability to understand visual information. Fluctuations in cognition, attention or alertness; Problems with movement including tremors, stiffness, slowness and difficulty walking; Visual hallucinations (seeing things that are not present); Sleep disorders, such as acting out one's dreams while asleep; Behavioral and mood symptoms, including depression, apathy, anxiety, agitation, delusions or paranoia; Changes in autonomic body functions, such as blood pressure control, temperature regulation, and bladder and bowel function. (Lewy Body Dementia Association, Inc.)

Our resident had many of these symptoms. When being changed at night, he would regularly raise his fists, swing his arms and try to kick us. He had lost total bowel and bladder function. The ability to understand what we were doing or why was lost on him. His body had become thin, emaciated, and yet he maintained superior strength. This is quite common with those with dementia. Once he had gotten a grip on me, it was very difficult to pull away.

One of his many problems was extreme stiffness brought on by his Parkinson's. At 4:00 am, when we needed to change his pad he could offer no help. His body had become rigid with his arms and legs stiffened. He could not bend his leg at the knee or his arm at the elbow. When he struck out, he did so using the full length of his legs and arms. Thus, it was very difficult to work with him. Over the years, I received several blows from him. My partner was not excused the punishment. But we carried on. It was our job.

Someone unknown and obviously unfamiliar with Lewy Body had the habit of raising the head of the bed to about 30 degrees. They would then place three pillows under his head. I estimated that his head was about 60 degrees, an impossible angle. He would slide down his bed, leaving his body flat with his head at that acute angle.

The addition of three pillows pushed his chin into his chest. Muscles, tendons and ligaments were overstretched. They were becoming atrophied (dying, fixed). Conversely, those at the front of his neck were constricting. If he were kept in this position, he would lose the use of his neck muscles.

I had to lower his head to a much more comfortable angle. This would reduce the already impaired movement of his neck. The procedure I adopted was long and tedious and often challenging. My first task was to lower the head of the bed to its lowest position. Because of the contraction of his neck, his head would stay where it was, hovering over his pillows.

It would take five to ten minutes for his head to settle into the pillows. After a few minutes, I would move one of the pillows. I would wait a further five or ten minutes before I could remove the second pillow. It would take almost thirty minutes before I had my resident resting on one pillow with his bed at the neutral position. His legs I kept resting on two pillows. Fluid build-up in lower limbs is a concern with someone sitting in a wheelchair for many hours. Raising those legs on a pillow or two is the correct procedure for reducing risks associated with this type of occurrence.

I raised the issue of the care given him by the previous shift to the nurse. I informed her of the way my resident was found in similar positions each shift. It was annoying. I told her that I believed his health was being compromised. I further stated that nothing in his chart suggested he should be put to bed and left in the position found. I told her that I believed it was not abuse, but cruelty. As usual, my complaint fell on deaf ears for nothing was ever done.

One very difficult night both my partner and I went into the resident's room to check his night brief. It was 4:00 am, the time for a full pad change as required by the inflexibilities of our night routine and the autocratic ruling of our night nurse. We found our resident lying in his urine and diarrhoea. His pad had become so congested that the accumulation of urine and liquid faeces had leaked past the edges of his pad and onto his bedding. His undershirt was saturated with his waste. The sight was bad, the smell even worse.

He was not checked for breathing at 2:00 am because we had an emergency that took time to resolve. Afterwards, we decided to wait the forty-five minutes for the round to begin.

Our resident was wearing his undershirt instead of the regular hospital style nightgown. We suspect that he put up a fight with the evening crew when he was being readied for bed. Instead of fighting with him, they put him to bed fully clothed. This was not unusual. We had often found him in similar circumstances. It was not uncommon to find others in this state. It made our care more difficult. But we had perseverance; along with a little stupidity.

He could no longer speak. His Parkinson's had left his vocal cords paralysed. We believed he could hear. Everything we did with him was explained to the fullest and extra time was allowed for each action of his care. However, it was quite clear he was afraid of falling out of bed. I would often tell him that everything was okay and that if he fell he would fall on me. He would have a soft landing. I was never sure if he understood. And he always fought us.

Although the smell in the room was nauseating, both my partner and I refused to wear a face mask. We hoped this would help to calm him. When we turned him, he became very anxious. Anxiousness quickly turned to anger. And anger resulted in fists and legs flying in the air as he tried to rid us of him. He was full of liquid faeces, and we desperately tried to avoid becoming contaminated.

We quickly took control of arms and legs. After easy removal of his soiled pad and soiled bedding, we tackled his undershirt. It was so badly sodden with human waste that it was glued to him like a second skin. I damned the evening shift. They had failed the resident. They had failed us. He should have been in a nightgown. And even though he would still be full of faeces and urine, it would have been much easier on him removing the gown.

To have to care for him in this manner was undignified, cruel. It was an injustice. His independence was no longer. His reliance on care was complete. He could do nothing by himself. He could neither call out for help nor press a call bell. And for some staff to allow this to happen is, without a doubt, unconscionable.

Removing his undershirt became a frightful task. We needed to sit the resident up. It was a task made even more difficult due to his Parkinson's disease. He was board-like, stiff. As he was unable to bend, I had to put my arm around his back and lever him up. I couldn't get him to sit upright; it just was not humanly possible. But I did get him to a position where my partner could start to pull his undershirt up. For five long minutes, we tried to get the shirt off him, but it became an impossible task.

We got his cold, foul smelling undershirt as far up his back as we could before it became immovable. Dreading the silent killer, hypothermia, I put a warm blanket around him while we discussed the next move. We could not save the shirt. The only way was to cut it off.

We were always reluctant to destroy clothing. Many nursing home residents have limited finances with a majority living on a fixed income. So impoverished are some that their clothing is in tatters. Buttons missing, zippers broken and holes in socks and undershirts are many of the late in life indignities they suffer. This was in our thoughts as discussions continued. The resolution appeared obvious. It was a solution that we were both loath to take.

I returned from the nurse's supply room with a pair of scissors. Rolling the resident on his side once again, I took the shears and ran them up his back, cutting the shirt from him. With the soiled, wet undershirt removed we could cleanse the resident. We quickly washed off the faeces and urine. We liberally applied a skin lotion to his entire body. Not only did the lotion protect his puckered skin but it had a pleasant fragrance. Had this been a rare occasion then mentioning it would not have had merit. Unfortunately, it wasn't. The situation had occurred many times. Fortunately, the other times it had occurred resulted in him being soaked in urine. And although that was problematic, it was a little easier to undertake.

Our request for proper care for our resident was simple and straightforward. We wanted him properly dressed for bed. We wanted his T-shirt and pants removed. We also wanted him dressed in a nightgown. It was agreed that this, and only this, would not only correct matters but also return a little dignity to him. There was no doubt in our minds that this alone would cut down on the difficulty we all too often faced. We believed that if the evening shift utilised the correct procedure, then the aggression shown would be substantially reduced.

It was not a major request. We were not asking any more of the evening shift than to do their jobs, and properly. We hoped the night RN would raise the issue with the evening shift and particularly with the LPN. Either this did not happen, or the evening LPN and staff chose to ignore the directive. Whatever the case, the resident would have to face the same unjust indignities many, many more nights.

On April 23, 2015, my resident passed away. I was not made aware of it until May 22, 2015. The investigator gave me a copy of his obituary. I remember well the smirk on his face as he handed it over to me. The resident's obituary was indeed glowing. One part of it reads:The family of (name deleted) wishes to express their sincere appreciation for the wonderful, compassionate care he received during the four years he spent at the nursing home. From all the staff, he received the ultimate care and attention, and for that, we are truly grateful. We feel so fortunate that he was treated with dignity and respect at all times and all staff was extremely supportive to his family.

The investigator took it upon himself to interview the resident's grieving widow and daughter (or close friend). I was taken aback. I now understood him. He would stop at nothing to find the proof he needed to disprove my allegations. I was not annoyed at him; rather, I was saddened for him. For someone to stoop so low as to interview those that had so recently lost a loved one was a callous act.

It took some seconds to gather my thoughts. When I did, I told him that everything that happened occurred at night. I told him that the resident's family was not there at 4:00 am. They were not privy to his nocturnal care. He could not speak. His disease had made him mute. The only communication about his care was from staff. And his family never saw or spoke to night staff. I then blurted out: "Had they been there at night and witnessed that of which I charted, I'm convinced they would not have written such a glowing tribute."

I felt the wrath of this man. The investigator had gone too far. He could have interviewed my partners and the duty RN to discover the truth. He could have obtained the legitimacy of my account by reading the residents charts. Instead, he took the word of a grieving widow who could not have known the truth. How could she?

I believe he raised the spectre of a lie by not telling the resident's wife the whole truth. After all, how could anyone give such a glowing report had they known what their loved one had gone through? It was a ploy by the investigator. But I wasn't finished with this resident, not yet, not by a long shot.

Night staff were required to deliver suppositories to those residents who were not ambulatory. It was a simple task. At 6:45 am we stopped getting residents up for the day and started delivering suppositories. Due to his Parkinson's disease, our resident's bowels had failed to work. Therefore, he was put on a bowel care programme that consisted of oral therapy and suppositories.

His doctor had ordered glycerine suppositories for him. This type of suppository provides a lubricant to the lower bowel to aid in expulsion of faecal matter. Each resident had their personal bowel chart. By date, the chart indicates if the resident had a Bowel Movement, what type (diarrhoea, loose, regular, constipated, etc.), how much faecal matter was produced and whether medication was used.

As he was bedridden, night crew were responsible for giving our resident his suppositories. After day three of no bowel movement, he was given his first suppository. There were no results. For the next five days, he received his early morning suppository. And still, there were no recorded results.

It became clear the suppositories had no effect. I discussed this with our nurse. She decided that it was time for a fleet enema. She placed the medication on the report table and wrote the resident's name on the box. As the night crew were not allowed to deliver the fleet enema, it was left up to days.

I was happy this positive step had been taken. It had been nine days since our residents last BM, and our collective minds turned to bowel impaction or twisted bowel. I began to question my resident's treatment. There are several different types of suppositories available each having a specific effect.

Dulcolax suppositories are a stimulant laxative. It acts directly on the bowels, stimulating the bowel muscles to cause a bowel movement.

Micro fleet enema. Colace Microenema is a stool softener. It works by adding water into the stool mass to soften the stool.

Fleet Enema contains sodium biphosphate and sodium phosphate. Each one is a form of phosphorus, which is a naturally occurring substance that is important in every cell in the body. Sodium biphosphate and sodium phosphate rectal is a combination medicine used in adults and children to treat constipation and to clean the bowel.

I had purposefully told the day crew about the resident's bowel history. And I pointed to the Fleet enema package put out for him. Whether they listened to me, I could not tell. The room was full of cackling female Care Aides. What I do know is that they failed to deliver the medication for when I returned that night for my shift, the medication was still on the desk.

I checked the resident's BM chart. There had been no entry. The previous day nurse told me that they had forgotten about giving him an enema. It had completely slipped their minds.

On March 26, 2015, I had a meeting with management. I informed both the Director of Care and the Assistant Director of Care of abuse. I cited the case of the resident going nine days without a BM and the cavalier attitude of his care staff. I was told that they had investigated and had found that a Care Aide had forgotten to chart that the resident had a BM. They told me that a correction was made in the resident's chart.

During the investigation, I was shown the resident's bowel chart. I was asked if I could see if a correction had been made during the nine days in question. I could see neither an entry of correction being made nor initials indicating one. Management had deceived me. I had been told a lie. They had tried to cover-up their failure. Perhaps they tried to stop me from raising the issue. I felt cheated. A pit in my stomach had opened up, leaving me nauseous. The knives were out, and I felt the urge to fight on dwindling.

The abuse of my resident was complete. And I had proven that nobody cared.

And we were only at day one of the investigation.

HYPOTHERMIA. THE SILENT KILLER

She was an elderly resident. Very thin, wiry. Her skin was very thin, delicate, almost translucent. Unkempt Salt and pepper hair curled chaotically. It gave little clue of its true length for when it was brushed, the bird's nest like clump stretched past her shoulders.

Her eyes sparkled with the mischievous flirtation only memories of youth could reveal. At her stage of dementia, those memories were gone, forever. But she still maintained the ability to focus on her care aides, especially when pleading for help, which, in later stages of her life, was often.

Her face was a forest of wrinkles, each a chasm plummeting deep into her pale greying skin. And without teeth, those wrinkles deepened as she wrapped her chin up and over her upper jaw. She would then busy herself chewing on her toothless gums. She had a wonderful face, and in her own way, she was beautiful. I never stopped telling her so.

When she first arrived on the unit she was generally pleasant, but she did have the ability to curse and loudly. She also reserved the right to strike out and at the most inopportune time. Punching and kicking were her favourite actions. We were always prepared for them. A swift kick to the mid-section, a punch on the arm or, as I quickly learned her speciality a good set of scratches down the arm.

I have lost count of the many scratches I received from her claw-like fingernails. And yet through all this I admired her. Her tenacity for self-preservation was insurmountable. It was midnight. My partner and I were doing our first nightly breathing check. As I glanced in the room I saw that our resident was laying on her right side facing away from me. Her bedclothes were crumpled up and on the floor. She had removed the bottom sheet, taken off her nightgown and pad and was curled up in a fetal position at the head of the bed. It was not uncommon to find her this way. Anytime she was upset or anxious we would find her in this state. However, the strong smell of urine wafting from her room gave me cause for concern.

I entered the room only to find my residents bed swimming in urine. With no bedding to soak up the liquid, it pooled on the mattress; a lagoon of urine. Her feet were resting in the ice-cold liquid. When my partner arrived, I was trying to get the resident away from a pool of urine. As much as I was trying to help my resident the more she fought me. It took the strength of my partner and I to move our resident onto the dry part of her mattress. And as we worked with her she kept on calling out, "I'm cold nurse, so cold." It was usual for her to cry out. During the later stages of her life she would call out for her son. Sometimes it would last the entire shift. Tonight, however, her shouting was tempered with shivering. I was deeply concerned for her health. The subtle signs of hypothermia were starting to manifest itself.

Hypothermia is that insidious chill that can take hold of the body and skewer it before anyone becomes consciously aware of it. Elderly frail people are far more vulnerable to it. Wasting muscle and paper thin skin fail to retain sufficient body heat. The larger surface area of skin on the adult causes greater evaporation, add to the mix a breeze from the air handling system, and the recipe for a slow, painless death is at hand. As an Emergency Medical Technician and a fascination for the malady I, perhaps, understood the risks more so than others. As soon as I realised the risks were in play, action was taken.

Everything had to be done in order. Get her dry was priority. That would slow evaporation; it would begin to slow the body's cooling, hypothermia. As soon as the mattress was relatively dry we began to assemble the clean bed linen. Placing clean linen on a bed with a hypothermic dementia resident is a battle royal. Great care and determination must be taken to avoid becoming annoyed at the resident. But that was our job, one of those jobs other care aides rarely saw.

Night shift was a permanent shift. Day and evening staff rarely, if ever, performed skills required by night staff.

When our residents bedding had been set, I left my partner to put her clean nightgown on. I walked briskly to the tub room and returned with a warm blanket.

Our resident had begun to settle. She was dry, her pad was dry. Her uncontrolled shivering had ceased. I placed the warm blanket directly on her. She responded with her normal whispered "Oh this is so nice." It signalled her slow return to normalcy. Her happy voice and gummy smile echoed her old self as she snuggled into the warmth.

She must have been exhausted for she quickly fell into a deep sleep. We heard neither hide nor hare from her for the rest of the night. I checked in on her every half hour until I was satisfied she was out of danger from that silent killer.

Had it been a rare occurrence it would have not been mentioned. My partner and I would have continued with little abatement. However, It was not rare to find residents extremely wet early in the shift. It should not happen. Residents wear night pads which can hold up to eight hours of urine, hence the name night pad. A care Aide can generally tell when the resident was last changed. It really wasn't rocket science. Finding our resident in such a condition, and many times throughout the year, drew suspicion of an uncaring Care Aide(s).

I had raised my concerns with the nurse. I told her that I could not understand how anyone could be so wet less than two hours after being checked. The evening crew were required to check all the residents during final 10:30 pm rounds. I didn't believe those rounds were ever done. After all, how could a situation like this occur. I hoped she would take up the challenge and find out why this was happening. As far as I know this did not happen for the cruel treatment continued unabated.

The term cruelty first raised it's ugly tone this night.

Cruelty would run neck and neck with abuse.

ALWAYS SHORT STAFFED

A reporter I was acquainted with sent me an email. He thought it appropriate. The document was of the 2013 Tours Report. CEO's from various Long Term Care facilities fanned out across the province, critiquing other facilities. A report would then be written to the Health Department and, presumably, corrective action would be taken. The idea was to determine problems within the Long-Term Care community and correct them. It, of course, never happened. CEO's and DOC's would throw their collective hands in the air crying they had insufficient funds to comply with the recommendations. Resident care would once again be held captive by the lack of money. If it was their way of attempting to blackmail the government into handing out extra funding, then either the government were not listening, or more to the point, they didn't care.

The truth that residents had been in bed and probably not turned for twelve hours looked back at me from those damning sheets. The resident council stated in 2013 that one resident was put to bed at 5:45 pm. He didn't get up until 9:00 am the next morning. To my utter sadness, the investigator refused to acknowledge that evidence. He stated that he held no credibility from the resident's council.

Family Councils Starter Kit - Terms of Reference

The main purpose of a Family Council is to improve the quality of life of residents and to give families and friends a forum for sharing their experiences, supporting each other, learning and exchanging information.

Family Council Membership A Family Council is a self-led, autonomous group. A Family Council develops its own Terms of Reference, including who may be a member. The Council may set provisions within its Terms of Reference for continuing the membership of a Family Council member who no longer has a family member/friend who is a resident in that home. This means that, while the wording of a specific Family Council mission or purpose statements may vary, many tend to be similar in focus. For example, regardless of the type of Home, its location or size, most Family Council mission statements identify all family members and friends as members, address the difficulties that many families encounter in the Special Care Home environment, and are committed to monitoring and increasing the well-being of the residents.

The main purpose of a Family Council is to improve the quality of life of residents and to give families and friends a forum for sharing their experiences, supporting each other, learning and exchanging information (family council pamphlet)

I showed the investigator the report from 2014. He became aggressive. He knew what was coming and he couldn't avoid it. The 2014 CEO's Tours report was a virtual carbon copy of the 2013 report. It was clearly damning. It was solid proof that nothing had been done in the twelve months preceding 2014.

A newspaper report positioned the CEO of the Health Regional directly in line with my original allegation of short staffing. This report also puts the government and the Health Minister on the firing line. They must have known these two reports were available. And when the Premier stood in the Legislature and intimated that there was no shortage of staffing, he clearly should have known that was just not the case.

The article was clear, unabashed. The president and chief executive officer of the Health Regions took full responsibility for the CEO Tours Reports. He said that he was disappointed, frustrated and that the action taken (or not, in this case) was not appropriate.

Except for a few minor additions and one elimination (the gentleman who was in bed for twelve hours), both reports were identical. The NDP labelled it a lazy government report. They said it was a cut and paste text from year to year, from facility to facility. The president and CEO of the health care region accepted the criticism, stating that he was the sole person accountable for this failure.

The SHRA CEO tried to paint a picture of his COE's touring the Health Region's nursing homes gathering data. He said that the idea was to talk to residents, families, and staff. The plan was to get CEO's out of their offices, to stop them looking at reports and statistics written by someone else. He was trying to get to the root of the problem, he said, believing he could get the proper answers to correct the problems.

I had already identified the problems and had come up with a reasonable fix. The problem was no one heard me except, of course, the staff and management I worked with. And they were not about to force issues that would show them in a bad light.

I told the investigator that the CEO of Saskatoon Health Care Region agreed with my findings. He agreed there was short staffing where I worked. So, I surmised, short staffing must lead to a reduction in health care standards. That reduction in standards means that those residents were being left for up to twelve hours without any physical attention. That was neglect, and neglect on purpose is abuse. "After all," I said, "you have to believe it, he's your boss. He signs your pay cheque."

Even though it was not over, not by a long shot, for now, I relished in the fact that I had the top dog in the Saskatoon Health Region agreeing with me. We were short staffed. No one in management at Oliver Lodge could disagree.

Management obviously cared little about the load factor of their staff. That gave the impression management cared little about their residents. If truth be known, not one person appeared to care. Not one iota.

"It was proof positive," I said without conviction. "Management knew that people were not being changed for at least six hours and in some cases up to twelve hours. Little was done to change the situation. It proved to me management just didn't care."

The investigator asked me if I'd considered going to the executive director about my complaints.

"What was the point?" I countered. I surmised that the executive director controlled the purse strings. Management had always laid the blame on lack of funds. It is an assumption, but I have to believe management approached him for an increase in their department budget. There was no extra money in that budget, so they constantly told us. If management couldn't get money for extra staff, what was the likelihood our argument would carry any weight? It's a fair bet our concerted argument would have been a waste of time. Besides, we met the CEO only once at our meetings. He was aloof, disassociated and seemed uncaring about his staff and residents alike.

I well remember a sign posted on a weekend schedule; from Friday shift through to Monday morning no overtime was to be allowed. That embargo on overtime included Care Aides, LPN and RN. To staff, it was proof positive budgets were running dry. The money would be saved on the backs of staff and residents alike. We would not be able to provide the care needed. We certainly could not provide the standard of care expected (if ever that standard was reached at night).

We did not hear from our union over the issue. We were on our own, to muddle through eight hours as best we could and to hell with any Standard of Care. It was, of course, almost criminal; but I'm sure not one person from management lost any sleep over the crisis. And as far as my employer's masters, the Health Region? Silence. I can't help but wonder if any other Long Term Care facility ever came under the same restrictions.

One weekend a dangerous short staffing situation arose when a Care Aide and an LPN failed to show. The overtime restriction was in play. I can only assume the two people phoned in sick. The rules stated that they were to inform management several hours before their shift. On an ordinary day, this would allow scheduling to find replacements. But this was night shift. On any regular night, We were overloaded with work. This night was to become a dangerous workplace.

With those two people, out of the picture, we had five Care Aides and one RN for 139 residents. It became a logistical nightmare. The RN organised staffing as best she could. One Care Aide was left on each of the four units. The spare Care Aide floated throughout the building helping as much as possible. The RN worked all units and was constantly running between floors. It was organised chaos. Fortunately, we got through the shift with little difficulty. However, it could have been a disaster had it not been for the fact that all those working were full-time staff.

The ratio of staff to resident appeared to be more than acceptable to management, giving rise to fears that this would become the norm. To my knowledge, the families of dementia residents were never informed of the pathetic situation.

Thoughts turned to lessons learned. Reduce the workforce and increase productivity: that is the goal of any business, and almost to a one, long-term care facilities are businesses. Reducing the workforce increases profit in two ways. It's logical and effective. We had inadvertently proven that we could successfully run the entire night operation with six people instead of eight. The loss of an LPN and a Care Aide would be substantial insofar as wages were concerned. This, of course, would bolster the facilities profits. We genuinely feared this would become a new level of staffing for nights. It didn't, but I'm sure the thought ran through management's fervent money hungry minds.

Although the investigator understood the process for complaints (he had been a manager of a nursing unit, after all), I decided to apprise him of my knowledge of the protocols for such matters. I just wanted to let him know that I was no dummy, that I understood the rules.

My role was to inform the duty RN of the issues I was facing on dementia. If she could not find a solution to the problem, then she would seek help from the Assistant Director of Care. If a resolution still could not be found, then she would look to the Director of Care for assistance. If still no decision was forthcoming, then the Chief Executive Officer would be asked to help. If the problem were financial, then he would approach the Board of Directors. The buck, as the expression goes, stops there.

The following was not known to me before the investigation. However, it must have been known to the investigator.

ROLES AND RESPONSIBILITIES (SHRA POLICIES & PROCEDURES) Number: 7311-10-003

Title: SPEAKING-UP - PROTECTION OF PERSONS REPORTING WRONGDOING

4.1 Vice Presidents, Executive Directors, Directors, Managers and Supervisors

4.1.1 Promote a positive and ethical work environment.

4.1.2 Ensure control measures are implemented within respective departments to prevent and detect wrongdoing.

4.1.3 Hold all suspected wrongdoing information received in the strictest confidence.

4.1.4 Ensure that the suspicion of a wrongdoing is reported.

4.1.5 Promptly advise the Vice President, People Strategies of complaints/concerns from employees regarding experiencing reprisal, for having made a report of wrongdoing or having participated in an investigation of wrongdoing.

Directors/Managers/Supervisors

4.3.1 Review all reports received of suspected wrongdoings and forwards the alleged incident to the appropriate department (e.g.(sic) Risk, Privacy and Compliance, OH&S, Security, *Labour Relations)*.

I discovered that I had followed the correct procedure. I had detected a wrongdoing (4.1.2). I reported the wrongdoing to the duty RN (4.1.4). Management, however, failed in their duty to promptly advise the Vice President, People Strategies of complaints/concerns from employees regarding experiencing reprisal, for having made a report of wrongdoing or having participated in an investigation of wrongdoing (4.1.5). They then failed to report to the appropriate departments (4.3.1). Had they followed the correct procedure I would not have faced an investigation. I would not have faced the distinct possibility of termination. And litigation would be the farthest thing from my mind.

I did what I was supposed to do. Management didn't.

I suspected there was a cover-up happening.

The corruption of silence was in play.

THE ULCER, AGAIN

I don't remember much about the early days of this resident. She was ambulatory and never caused us any problems. Her sleeping habits were excellent and thus, I hardly ever saw her. However, she was an early riser and became one of the group of regulars on our early coffee and cookie round table.

She was slight, yet tall. She had wispy, ethereal hair that drained over her shoulders to come to rest at her waist. It wasn't salt and pepper, and yet it wasn't white. I was never one for getting her hair properly brushed and putting it in a bun or pigtail. It was something I just could not do. Other staff would have to put the stringy mane in a ponytail or perhaps a braid.

Her skin had the look of leather, a testament to a life of hard work. And yet her skin was also very fragile, paper-thin, and would bruise or tear with the trifling of a careless touch. We had to be careful with her. Our touch was always specific and gentle. Carefully we cleansed her and readied her for the day.

She had her own teeth. And as much as we would have liked to keep them healthy it became impossible. As with most dementia residents, she would clamp down hard on the toothbrush. We had to watch as her teeth rotted.

I do not remember if at any time she did not wear a skirt and blouse. On Sundays, we would dress her in an ankle length dress. I had always believed Sunday a special day, a day to dress up a little more than the rest of the week.

At first, she could communicate with ease. Although short-term memory is impaired, dementia residents can search back in time and remember long ago memories. She was no different. Being born in the early 1920's and to a farm family, she often talked about hardship and hard work. The youngest of nine siblings with five of them brothers didn't spare her the rigours of early rise and chores in the barn. After, she would have to walk a five-mile hike to school. She relished in stories of her mother teaching her how to cook on a coal and wood stove.

It was her trek to school that shone through her eyes. It was something she must have enjoyed for she spoke of it often. In the summer, walking the grid road to town, kicking up dust and throwing small stones as far as she could. Then in the winter, bundled up and facing winds and an ambient temperature of minus thirty degrees. She couldn't remember if she ever stayed away from school, either from sickness or extreme cold. She must have been a trooper. I know that she was the last surviving member of her family, parents and siblings all paving the way for her and I secretly hoped she would find them again.

As with all dementia residents, as death approached she became bed-ridden. We had been changing her every night at four in the morning, frequently finding her very wet and occasionally needing to change her bedding. More importantly, she could not move by herself. Pressure point injury was a distinct possibility as its slothful journey to skin eruption began.

My resident met all the prerequisites of probable skin breakdown. She was bedridden and couldn't move. Her skin was constantly wet. Her head was raised to thirty degrees without warrant. She lay on turning sheets. It was these sheets and her head at thirty degrees that would eventually give rise to me saying that she had been abused.

I had learned early on that dementia residents often showed little or no response to pain. Pain in the throes of death, however, is a different matter. It was a phenomenon that raised its ugly head teaching each of us a patent lesson in dementia care.

A situation occurred a year or two prior that makes a strong point. About 1:00 am a resident walked to the nursing station complaining of blood on her nightgown. She was not cognitive. But it was clear she was unhappy with her bloodied nightdress. She had always been prim and proper, and dirty nightwear obviously caused her concern.

She had injured a finger. That was the cause of her bloodied nightgown. She had what appeared to be a dislocated small finger with the joint breaking through the skin at the second joint. There was no sign of her being uncomfortable with her finger.

I was aware that my bedridden resident was in danger of attaining ulcers as she could no longer move in bed. As per routine prescribed by the nurse, I was not allowed to turn or change any resident until 4:00 am. I decided that the risk for ulcers was so great that I needed to break the rules. I unquestionably became proactive, to turn and change residents that required it at 2:00 am irrespective if I had help or not. Most often I did not have any assistance. Residents were once again turned at 4:00 am. My resident became part of this group. Turning her at both 02:00 and 04:00 am helped to avoid debilitating pressure on her coccyx and hips.

Through the summer and up to Christmas of 2014 she remained clear of any ulcers. Between December 16, 2014, and January 2015, I did not work due to poor health.

Before returning to work, my wife had scolded me for turning and repositioning residents by myself. One never argues with one's wife over such matters, so I did as I was instructed. I followed the Dementia Care Aide routine to the letter.

My residents were returned to their routine of being changed and turned at 4:00 am. From January 2015 to March 26, 2015, I was aware that other Care Aides had also adhered to the same routine. With this change, I was acutely aware that my resident would almost certainly develop ulcers on her coccyx.

Due to an injury, on April 1, 2015, I was placed on day shift and light duties. It was a rare occasion that I would see my residents in the daylight and wearing normal clothing.

On April 07, 2015, I found myself in the dementia unit. It was lunchtime. I was asked to feed my resident as she could not feed herself. It was a nice change, for working nights I rarely had the opportunity to assist residents with their meals. With my spirits high I went to her room carrying a tray of food for her.

During my years as a Care Aide, I had always sung and whistled. Today was no exception. Even though I was under a cloud of suspicion (something of which I was unaware) I continued my crooning. I had a skip in my step, and I looked forward to assisting my resident.

When I reached her room, I learned what had happened to her over the previous few months. She had developed a large third-stage ulcer on her coccyx. I wasn't surprised. I knew it would happen. It was a simple case of the nurse not understanding, or refusing to understand, the insidious way ulcers attack the body. To this day I believe it was a total lack of commitment by nursing staff to ensure the proper standard of care was given to all residents.

It was a simple case of the nurse believing she knew best. It also seemed an unpretentious case of management standing back, understanding but doing nothing. 'The routine must be followed,' was the cry no matter the consequences. In this case, the consequences were dire.

At night dementia residents had their care delayed to accommodate staff meal breaks. All other residents in the facility had their care done, including pads changed, where necessary and, of course, turned before meal breaks. It was only in dementia that proper care would have to wait until 4:00 am. In dementia, it was a case of staff first, residents second.

Management was quick to realise by using the posted routine; their budget would be spared the extra expense of employing another Care Aide. Without a doubt the CEO was happy. Likewise, the board would also be pleased. The nurse, who seemed to cower under the scrutiny of the ADOC, accepted the status quo with little comment. My advocacy for my resident had been covered-up by all those so-called experts. I was despondent. The resident, regrettably, was the one that suffered. Her damning ulcers could have been prevented if only someone had cared. But that was the problem. No one seemed to do so.

I tried to feed her, but her mouth remained closed. No matter how I encouraged her to eat, she would turn away. Refusal was all she understood. She was heading for death. The ulcers made that journey shorter. I had warned so many staff that this would happen. My protestations had fallen on deaf ears. That spectre of ignorance once again raised its ugly head, and I was left to witness the result of my premonitions.

There was nothing I could do. The damage had been done, and there was no turning back. When two Care Aides arrived to turn her, she let out a soft moan. She felt pain, it was obvious. As with most Care Aides, they didn't understand the complexity of turning a body to reduce stress, and therefore pain.

In my other profession, emergency care workers understand the need to keep a body in alignment, to maintain rigidity. A minimum of three people is needed to turn a body. The spine must be kept in a straight line, to keep the body as immobile as possible. In Long Term Care the use of manpower to turn someone is left to two caregivers. One person on one side of the body while the other situates themselves on the other side. Using specially treated sliding sheets the resident is both pulled and pushed to one side of the bed. Turning then occurs. The body is turned half way and comes to rest on its side. Work is then started. After completion, the resident is turned 180 degrees to their other side to complete the work. The resident is then placed in the appropriate position. Depending on the weight of the resident the procedure can be achieved without much difficulty. However, a tall or heavy resident presents serious problems not only for the resident but also for the staff.

No matter the weight of the resident, it is not possible to maintain a rigid spine utilising the procedure as outlined in TLR. That, unfortunately, is the price we pay for the lack of funding or ignorance.

The resident was tall, but not particularly heavy. Due to her length, the turn was difficult. Her head and mid-trunk turned without much difficulty. The lower trunk and legs, however, failed to turn with the rest of the body. It followed only after being pushed over by a staff member. The result was a twisting of the lower body at the top of the pelvis. The spine and ulcers were compromised with the ulcerations being further damaged by the involuntary twisting motion.

I could not put the blame on the two staff members for the improper manoeuvre. They knew no better. Their training did not reach into body mechanics and movement of injured people. That training went to Emergency unit nurses, ambulance personnel, to people like me and me.

Because of our ignorance, many, many Long Term Care residents suffer needlessly. This resident suffered needlessly.

I didn't see her again. She died while the investigation into abuse progressed. When I was informed of her death by the interrogator, I was upset. I told him that had she been turned every two hours as I had done, then she wouldn't have died that way and may have lived a longer life. I was told, and in no uncertain terms, that the resident's physician did not agree with me. I asked when it was her doctor visited her. "Did he examine her in the summer and fall of 2014? Did he read her chart and thoroughly? Did he talk to her caregivers? Did he suggest that she should be turned every two or four hours"? Of course, I received no reply. To the investigator the doctor's opinion was sacred. In my view the doctor's opinion was wrong.

This resident died in part because of ulceration of her coccyx. It could have been prevented. I had warned the night staff of the probable outcome. Nothing happened with the resident's care.

    No one cared.

        Her nursing team didn't care.

            The system didn't care.

                She was abused, and I hang my head in sorrow.

THE WANDERER

Rooms in the new facility had high, twelve-foot ceilings. The windows were equally high, allowing for light to swim in and bathe the residents. The dining room and TV lounge ceilings had architecturally scrolled etchings embossed into the noise damping tiles.

Lighting was more than sufficient for all shifts. The only complaint was that the night lighting was too bright. It was bright enough to fill the cavernous hallways and to satisfy the most discerning of Care Aides. By and large dementia residents do not like bright light, I, therefore, found it strange that lights of this nature should have been put into a secure unit. But then this was a strange unit with silliness abound.

When the facility first opened, the walls were decorated with glass-covered pictures. Resident's history boxes were also covered in glass. Metal iron sculptures ornamented the walls of the small sunroom. There was also a fake ficus tree in the same room. Leather recliners were used in the TV lounge. Bedroom door handles were of the lever type and the closets, although locked, were simple to open by the resident. Only two of the thirty-two bedrooms could be seen from the nursing station.

It took less than two weeks for wandering residents to open other resident's doors. Doorknobs eventually replaced the lever handles. Even then a few residents manipulated the doorknob to gain access to the room (rarely their room). Plastic childproof handles were used to try and put a stop it to the entry. They worked relatively well with only two residents having the grip to gain entry. (One of those was my big teddy bear). The handles lasted over a year until one day they were removed. We never knew why. We can only surmise that somehow, someone deemed them illegal, probably from SHRA.

One resident was notorious for leaving her room after evening staff put her to bed. Therefore, to keep her in her room, staff put a childproof door handle on the inside doorknob. It worked. She could no longer get out of her room. The Care Aide who told me about the resolution to the problem appeared excited. She stated that they didn't have to deal with the resident anymore. "Put her in her room, and she stays there." What was done was wrong. It smacked of restraint, of a prison. It was not care; it was an abuse of power.In another incident of stupidity by the interior decorator, were glass framed pictures. They adorned the walls of the hallway that were invisible to night staff. One early morning a resident pulled one of the pictures down and placed it gently on a dining table. The picture measured four square feet. There were visions of glass being shattered and pieces used as missiles. Within a week all glass framed pictures had been removed and replaced with canvas ones. They were then secured to the wall at each corner of the picture.

And the metal ironwork in the sunroom? A resident ripped it from the wall and bent in three. Urinating on the Ficus tree became a popular sport for the residents. Although it was a fake tree, it eventually rotted away. The leather chairs were beautiful when new. But urine and faeces soon rotted them as well. As with the artwork and the tree, the chairs found the garbage bin.

It took three years, but eventually, a CCTV (closed circuit television) system was installed. This equipment allowed staff to observe wandering residents. We could see what was happening at night in each of the three hallways. The system had the ability to zoom in on the wandering resident. Unfortunately, staff were never trained to use the apparatus. This was the type of environment in which we were working. It was a disaster waiting for a bigger disaster.

New bathtubs had auto fill. Water temperature was also automatic. With a push of a button, the tub could be raised and lowered with ease.

On-board cleaning equipment made the stressful job of bathing a resident easier. It also helped reduce back injury.

Each tub room was equipped with a mobile lift to move the resident from their wheelchair to the tub. As usual, the lift came with small wheels that caused slight difficulty when pushing a large resident. Two Care Aides pushing and guiding the resident would overcome this difficulty. The lift came with a built-in weigh scale. Each resident's weight was recorded every month.

Along with recording weights, other information was also charted. Blood pressure, pulse, breathing and blood oxygen levels became the resident's monthly health check-up. The information gathered gave a continual map of the resident's welfare. Apart from recording the resident's weight, all other assessments were completed by the nurse.

Both tub rooms and the nursing supply room were equipped with a towel/blanket warmer. I purposefully ensured that every night that two blankets were in each. The warmers were not about to escape my criticism. The temperature of each should have been set to 120F. Care Aides felt that 120F was not warm enough. So they turned the warmers up. On one occasion I found a warmer with a temperature of 190F. Towels inside were scorching and extremely hot. No matter how many requests for maintenance to rectify the problem were written, nothing was ever done. I believe it's just a matter of time before a fire starts.

Each resident had a private room with a bathroom. Wardrobe space was plentiful with all wardrobe and cupboards lockable. One bedside table and three strange storage units on wheels and hidden under a window shelf complemented the spacious room. Some rooms came equipped with ceiling track lifts.

Most residents had the new TLR-style beds. These beds could be lowered to within four inches of the floor. These were given to residents who were most likely to fall out of bed. These rooms were equipped with fall-out mats. TLR states that there should be two mats, one on either side of the bed. Often this was not the case. Older beds were used for those residents who were ambulatory. Other beds were utilised for residents who were bedridden. This type of bed also utilised fall-out mats. Even though the resident was bedridden, it did not mean to imply they could not move.

The dementia unit was built as a square with the nursing station, two dining rooms, a kitchen and two television lounges on one of the walls while the other three held residents' rooms, linen closets, and bathtub rooms.

Night staff used to scratch our collective heads at the architecturally proven design. At no time could we see more than two resident's rooms from the nursing desk. Had it not been for the alarm system installed in each room, and later the CCTV system, we would not have been aware of any wandering residents.

The resident alarm system consists of multi-sensors, all filtering through a computer program and then to a pager to alert the Care Aide: Bed sensor: A narrow sensor strip four inches wide and as wide as the bed. It is placed at the resident's shoulders at the upper of three joints of the bed. The strip is placed directly on the mattress underneath the bed sheets. Should the resident move off the sensor (as in, getting out of bed), an audible alarm will be triggered on the Care Aides' pager. Bathroom sensor triggered when someone enters the bathroom. Again, this was displayed on the Care Aide's pager. Door sensor activated when the resident exited and entered the room. A wander-guard bracelet, worn by each resident in dementia, which would lock all exit doors if they moved too close.

Care Aides, the duty nurse, and the LPN were required to carry a pager. It showed real-time information such as room number, what alarm had been triggered, the time it was triggered and other unexplained gibberish that often appeared on the screen.

When the alarm system worked, it afforded amazing results. I could sit at the nursing station and follow a resident's whereabouts. I could even track him when he left his room and whether he entered another resident's room or not. It was unfortunate both the LPN and RN failed to carry their respective pagers. They complained bitterly that the pagers would go off throughout the night. Their quiet was being disturbed. It was a sham.

When the system worked, it worked very well. Unfortunately for the first three years, it didn't.

The alarm system was under tight control of the CEO and his head of maintenance. Both had ultimate control. It was their pride and joy. The CEO had never used the system, ever. And yet when things went wrong each feigned ultimate knowledge, for it was their Baby.

When things went wrong (and they did, and often), they always denied the system was at fault. They told us that it was the user who was at fault. We didn't know how the system worked. Instructions for its use were at a minimum. It was a learn as you go exercise. It was stupid. This little apparatus was our direct link to our residents, and our knowledge of how and why it worked was kept as a secret by the CEO.

Many memos with instructions on how to fix the situation filtered through the report room. It became nauseating. I suggested that perhaps we could have the system checked by the original installers. That idea failed, almost certainly by management to preserve what budget they had left.

I found it extraordinarily strange that after complaining for nearly three years about the systems failures, no one from maintenance or, for that matter, the CEO, would show up on the night shift to witness for themselves their baby's failure.

For three years, the nurse had been sending emails to both these gentlemen. They were constantly informed of the alarm system failures. They were told that sometimes it would work and yet other times, it wouldn't. Sometimes we could understand what was on the screen, other times it was gibberish. The truth was, it was unreliable. And management's answer to our questions became more silly as time went on.

This stupid nonsense of "not our problem but yours" carried on for several years. That was until, one day when the system went berserk. I was receiving alarms every ten to fifteen seconds. They were coming so fast I was unable to clear the pager of the backlog of calls. Within two hours I shut my pager off.

We sent an email to both 'owners' explaining the phenomenon. Instructions were returned via a memo advising us what to do to correct the situation. That night it took only one and a half hours for me to threaten to throw the pager out the window. The nurse agreed. And again, an email was sent to the owners. And again, an email returned stating that there was nothing wrong, smarten up, suck it up, use the thing properly. I understood that silliness had stopped. Stupidity had replaced it.

I was becoming extremely frustrated. Being told it was our fault was ridiculous in its extreme. I felt as though we were being made scapegoats for inept management. Then I found that little chink in their collective armour. It would destroy their frustratingly silly attitude.

That night, and after only half an hour with the most hated malfunctioning device, I checked the calls history. We had a monitor in the unit report room. It displayed every call the pager received, and then some. Sure enough, it identified every call received during the previous night's shift. I showed the evidence to the nurse. I asked her to send an email to our 'dear friends' asking them to do one thing: check the history files.

Within two days the system was fixed. It never caused issues again. For three years, I had been complaining of the failure of the system. And for those years I was being told I did not know what I was talking about. Those in power claimed they did. They were proven wrong. One would have thought that an apology was in the offing. That these big men would cower just a little, and show their staff some respect. Of course, when one reaches the lofty heights of CEO, apologies are extremely rare. For us, his subservient, it did not happen.

I quickly realised that the word respect, which is raised at all levels of care, was never truthfully given from management. Respect of staff -- believing they had knowledge -- was not only dismal but in a lot of cases turned to disrespect. I would find out during the investigation that doctors, managers, nurses, LPN's and colleagues had little to no respect whatsoever. This, of course, included the investigator.

Lesson learned we moved on. Several years after the unit was opened a Closed-Circuit Television system (CCTV) was installed. The monitor was set on a high shelf. It had been placed in the very small report room. To watch it I had to tip my neck backwards at a 45-degree angle. Not very comfortable. And then we were never trained on the CCTV system, another of those management secrets of "tell 'em just enough". The monitor had been divided into four segments. Each segment showed one of three hallways.

It was easy to spot if someone had left their room. Our pagers triggered. And we could identify the resident. Unfortunately, the picture on the CCTV monitor was so small, identifying the resident was by trial and error. There was a way to enlarge the quarter picture to full screen, but we didn't know how. Ah! Those stupid secrets. Management, we assured ourselves, were complete boneheads.

Our superiors were distant and aloof. Contact, except the thirty-minute meeting with management every six weeks or so, was non-existent. And Care Aides stood far too low on the ladder to warrant any meeting with the CEO.

None of those in lofty heights bothered themselves with issues we were constantly raising. Headboards coming loose? Fix them yourself.

Blanket warmers too hot? Ho hum. Pagers not working? Heard it all before. By and large, any complaints or advice from any night staff was ignored.

We were getting nowhere with management on issues that were affecting us. However, that didn't stop me from raising the issue of neglect of my residents. For several months, beginning in 2014, I could see a rapid decline in the care of residents. When I started my shift, many were saturated in their urine, some wallowing in faeces. It was a common occurrence. I talked to the nurse about it, but as usual, I was ignored. At the monthly shift meetings, I received similar feedback: nothing.

We had been working short staffed for a long time. Indeed, in late 2013 we had been told that money had been found for extra staff. Nothing would materialise. We had to put up with what we had. It was my first indication management would say and do anything to appease us even though they knew they were speaking half-truths and innuendos.

In early March 2015 Cam Broten, leader of the opposition, was mentioned in a newspaper article. He was concerned about the staffing levels at a care home where he said that was a ratio of one staff to twelve residents. I smiled. I could have laughed, but I didn't. Instead, I quickly did the math. My figures were a damning testament to night shift Care Aides. I showed the article to the day crew. Smiles and laughter and "I wish we had it that good" were commonplace.

I sat on the article for two weeks pondering my fate and that of my residents.

THE FALL GIRL

She was a small but robust woman, one that had held life in her hands, took it by the throat, stepped into the battle and won. For forty years she had been a schoolteacher and by all accounts a good one. A photograph depicting her first one room school was pinned to her notice board. Several children were in front of the school. Although it was a paper photocopy the truest sense of the historical picture shone through.

The picture was full of pinholes. People had removed it from the corkboard and then put it back without using the same hole. I just hoped the original photograph was still in good condition and being looked after. It was not only a small part of her history but more significantly, a part of Saskatchewan history.

She lived in the present, but the present often lasted only five minutes. Even then she was kind and courteous to staff and other residents. Her good mornings were always spoken with a warm smile.

She remained submissive and was cooperative in all her care. But as her disease was wanton, passivity turned to antagonism. She became angry with staff. Where once her morning care could be done by one person, it now took two. And even then life was not easy. The odd punch or pinch would manifest itself without warning. An ever-watchful eye was always needed.

She was until I saw her last, ambulatory and could get to the toilet by herself. As usual, when her bed alarm triggered we would leave her for five to ten minutes before resetting it. We wanted to give her as much independence as possible. Independence was one of the most important achievements I could offer residents.

The workload placed on staff during the day is such they didn't have sufficient time to allow their residents that luxury of independence.

They had insufficient time to wait for a resident to get themselves dressed, shave, apply makeup, etc. I did not suffer that rigorous test. The night shift was required to get up four residents, two that were ambulatory and two who were non-ambulatory (those who required full lifts).

Early mornings were often busy. What with getting four residents ready for the day and then delivering suppositories for those who needed them, we tended to be rushed. Worse still was when we found several residents wandering. Safety first was our goal. So along with the prior work, we would often find ourselves getting a few more residents washed and dressed. But that was the job.

Nighttime was frequently as busy. One night at 1:26 am (as charted) my schoolteacher resident left her bed. As usual, I gave her a few extra minutes. At 1:40 am (taken from the alarm history) I cancelled the room alarm and entered. I found her on the floor a good ten feet from her bed. She was sitting in her urine. I quickly assessed the scene. I then called the nurse and my partner, telling each that there had been a fall. I then performed a primary and secondary assessment.

She was in a sitting position facing the bathroom. Her left leg was outstretched while the other was tucked under her. She was supporting herself with both hands behind on the floor. A skid mark of approximately three feet in front of her was clearly visible in the urine. It seemed clear to me she had slid down, not sat down. Injuries to her skeletal system were, as far as I was concerned, a distinct possibility.

Completing a secondary assessment, I assured myself there were no major injuries. I further assured myself that her neurological status appeared normal. Standing behind her and supporting her back I waited until help arrived. I was a little concerned about her coccyx and possible left hip as she had her right leg underneath her. I decided to wait until the nurse arrived to do a skeletal assessment.

Within five minutes both the nurse and my partner arrived both from different units. As usual, the nurse shouted to the resident, "Are you hurting anywhere?" There was no response. I advised the nurse of my concerns regarding possible coccyx and hip damage. There was no reaction. She decided, as normal, to get the resident dressed in the lift sling. The RN did not perform an assessment before manhandling the resident. I was alarmed. I had done my duty. I had told the nurse of my concerns. From that point on I accepted the RN's seniority. I did as directed.

As we moved the resident to put the sling on her, it became obvious that she had attempted to pull her pad down to urinate. She couldn't reach the toilet in time. Consequently, she had relieved herself on the floor.

I watched her face very carefully to see if there was any sign of pain. I was still very concerned about the real potential for damage to her spine and hips. To my relief there was none. When she was in her sling we moved the resident to her bed and began the challenge of removing her long-brushed cotton nightgown. And a challenge it most certainly was for most who fall become frightened and tend to fight Care Aides. She was no exception.

Wet clothes have a propensity to stick to people. As discussed earlier, we have had to cut clothing away from residents for this very reason. However, in this case, the resident stopped fighting once we got the offending article of clothing over her waist.

Around her waist and down her thigh was a night pad. It should not have been there. She was ambulatory. She could toilet herself. The pad she was wearing had four sticky tabs attached that held the pad in place. They were not made for the wearer to remove; rather they were designed for staff to remove.

The resident should have been wearing a pull-up. Like ordinary underwear, this incontinence product is designed to aid the resident when toileting herself. I had asked the evening crew to keep her in a pull-up for sleeping. I was ignored. It was becoming a common occurrence. It quickly became apparent evening staff believed they knew better. In their eyes, the night crew were of little consequence.

Had this been an isolated case then it would not even rate a footnote. But it wasn't. I could name at least six residents who went through the same process. The evening crew were made aware of each case, and in each one, our pleas for consistency in incontinence products for residents were totally ignored. It was a disaster waiting to happen. The evening crew failed to respond to our requests. On purpose? I do not know. But it appears they just didn't care.

After we had returned the resident to her bed, the nurse instructed me to chart the fall as a slide-out. She then left to return to her normal duties.

The resident survived, and free of injury, although she never regained the gumption to wander much anymore. Indeed, as I recall she became another resident that had lost part of her independence. She would become another that would have to be changed at night.

The nurse instructed me to chart the fall as a slide-out. A slide out occurs when a resident falls from her bed onto a fall out mat. This resident was ambulatory. When a resident can walk, they do not have fall-out mats. Besides, a slide-out cannot occur ten feet from the bed.

During this part of the investigation, I suggested, and strongly, that the RN did not take a full assessment of the resident; she did not take an initial vitals assessment; she did not check for any signs of injury to either skeletal or neurological systems; she did not return for the second vitals assessment. She failed in her duties, and completely.

Standard assessment procedure is to:
- ➢ Assess the resident from head to toe when he/she is found on the floor or seen falling and make sure it is safe to assist the resident to a chair before moving him/her.

- Not move the resident until it has been determined that nothing is broken or sprained.
- Take a full set of vital signs.
- Interview the resident and any witnesses to the fall to determine the exact circumstances and cause of the fall.
- After the assessment and treatment are done, notify the resident's responsible family member and physician of the incident.
- Adequate documentation in the nurses' notes and the incident report will include all the above.
- The occurrence should also be noted in the 24-hour report for follow-up monitoring, reports, and acute charting.
- The fall and its time, date, and location should be entered in the Falls Log.
- The facility's policy and procedure should give detailed guidelines for filling out incident reports. The nurse's notes must never state that an incident report has been filled out since this will allow possible litigation actions.
- The nurse has specific duties to perform post falls. It is one of her many tasks that must be completed.
- Post-fall protocols are clearly outlined for follow-up, documentation, and monitoring.
- Post- fall assessment is comprehensive.
- Guidelines indicate protocols for filling out and following through with incident reports.
- Medication review is done after fall.
- The facility's policy and procedure should clearly outline what actions are to be taken
- Immediately after a fall. It should also indicate what documentation is to be done.

> The incident report and nurse's notes should include the following information:
- The time and location of the fall
- Location of any injury
- Results of the head to toe assessment
- Vital signs
- The cause of the fall if known
- Treatment
- Post-fall interventions
- Statements made by the residents and any witnesses
- Time the family was notified
- Time the physician was notified
- New fall intervention implemented to prevent reoccurrence (sic)
- All Incident Reports must be turned into the Director of Nursing as soon as they are filled out by the nurse in charge. The Director of Nursing examines them for accuracy, making sure the resident's family and physician were informed of the incident, and that required follow-up charting is completed in the resident's chart. If there are nursing care plan issues related to the incident, they can be addressed in the next staff meeting. Incident reports are also reviewed and signed by the Administrator and Medical Director. They are kept in a file at the facility for several years.

The Post Fall Investigation is a fact-finding mission to discover the cause and eliminate it if possible. The goal is to prevent future falls. All of the resident's medications should be reviewed.

Changes made to the nursing care plan should include adding new interventions and the evaluation of the effectiveness of prior fall-prevention strategies.

I looked at the accident as any OHS safety investigator would (I am a certified OHS accident investigator). In any accident, the first question asked is: "What was the root cause?" followed by: "What triggered the accident? Could the accident have been prevented? Could the findings reduce/stop another accident?" All these questions saturated my mind as I sat at the nursing station, revisiting the scene and my observations. It wasn't long before I found the answers and it would be encapsulated in one short paragraph.

1. The root cause was the resident's need to use the bathroom.
2. The resident was wearing a full pad at the time.
3. Due to the complexity of undoing the full brief, it slipped from her waist on one side and ended up on her knees.
4. Unable to reach the bathroom in time, she urinated on the floor.
5. The resident slipped in her urine.
6. The resident fell to the floor on her coccyx and hips.
7. Conclusion: Had she been wearing the proper incontinent product she would probably have had sufficient time to reach the toilet. Therefore, the fall may not have occurred.

As for fault of the system? Nights will often ask the evening crew to ensure that specific tasks are completed for various residents. This request is never intended to lessen the workload of the night shift but more allowing the resident the best sleep they can get. This, in return, not only helps the day crew with a more compliant resident but it also helps the resident to stay awake during the day and to be more amicable to the care offered.

Communication between evenings and night crew do not exist. They had never existed. Our
nurse knew of this but did nothing to alleviate the problem. Management was also aware
of the ongoing situation but turned a blind eye. The problem festered. And as usual, residents and staff were mistreated, abused.

Our resident survived the fall. The investigator implied that I had lied. The nurse survived my accusation of wrongdoing. And yet the investigator told the union rep and me that no proper documentation existed in regards to the fall. In other words, the resident never fell. The nurse was never called to the room, and neither was my partner

What is interesting is the room alarm shows my arrival and departure time (when the alarm is brought back online). Closed Circuit Television should also have recorded those times as well. There is no doubt that within my scope of practice I should not have performed a primary and secondary assessment. Accordingly, it was within the nurse's scope of practice to perform both those assessments. I had been working with that nurse for four and a half years and had never known her to perform a complete assessment on any fallen resident. Indeed, I don't think I saw any nurse perform the correct procedure.

As soon as I got back to the nursing station I charted what I had seen and done. The RN charted about the fall at 3:00 am. No other documentation was ever done. As far as I'm concerned, the fall exists only in the resident's chart. I was happy to be told that the RN had followed me in charting that it was a fall.

A previous fall had befallen a resident. This time the resident was not wet nor was she trying to get to the bathroom. She had a habit of waking up about 1:00 am. She had a king-sized bedspread on her single bed. I had notified management of the danger of the very large bedspread as the resident carried it around with her, much like a child's baby blanket. I advised them that it would be a matter of time before she would trip on the material. This night she had reached her bedroom door before becoming consumed by the enormous bedspread and falling to the floor.

Again, I called the nurse and my partner. And again, we put the woman back to bed. And once more I was told to chart that it was a slide-out.

A word on slide-outs versus falls: The SHRA was gathering data on falls in all affiliated nursing homes. My employer's fall statistics were not as healthy as they should have been. All falls had been recorded and charted as they occurred irrespective of how or where they happened. It was something we could not control. Each resident had the right to get out of bed, and conversely, each resident had the right to fall, and if that fall injured the resident in any way, then that was considered unfortunate. That was the price of independence.

We had received instructions, via email, from management to alter our way of charting falls. On one shift the RN informed us that she had received an email stating that there had been to many reported falls. We were told that if a resident landed close to their bed on or off a fall mat, it must be charted as a fall-out. This type of fall would not generate a fall report. It would be charted as a simple slide out of bed. The RN would not be required to attend the resident unless there was a clear indication of injury. The Care Aides would perform primary and secondary assessments before lifting the resident back to bed. The nurse would be told about the slide-out before going off shift.

The slide-out would not show up on monthly statistics and would put my employer in good light.

The investigator didn't like me at this point. I was now suggesting that the nurse had been unprofessional in her duties. I was also suggesting that management were fraudulent in their obligations to SHRA. They hadn't done their respective duties. And I, a lowly Care Aide, was spilling the beans. He had tried to mire me in the aspects of my job. "Was I hired as a Care Aide or an EMT? Did I have the right to perform assessments"? And on and on. It was nauseating. I couldn't get it through his thick skull that the nurse didn't do any assessments. Had I not done them, as he suggested I should not have, and there was an injury to the resident, litigation would almost certainly result. And although he accepted the nurse did not do her job as per protocol, it was I who was facing the punishment.

THE POLITICAL STORM

I had had enough. No one at the Long-Term Care facility where I worked was listening to my complaints of abuse. I had used photographs to present my case to the duty RN. I had apprised management of my concerns many times. I had sought opinions from my many work partners. And as I brought forward my concerns at our monthly meetings with management, all failed to acknowledge the calamity some residents were going through. I knew I was on my own.

I needed to open Pandora's box. To let the secret out, to tell people, anyone who would listen, the ills that I was witnessing night after night. And so if management were not going to listen to me, then perhaps politicians would. And so my nightmare began.

FOURTH SESSION - TWENTY-SEVENTH LEGISLATURE
of the
Legislative Assembly of Saskatchewan

DEBATES
and
PROCEEDINGS

(HANSARD)
Published under the
authority of
The Hon. Dan D'Autremont Speaker
N.S. VOL. 57 NO. 42A MONDAY, MARCH 30, 2015, 13:30
part of Hansard
The Speaker: — I recognise the Leader of the Opposition.
Provision of Seniors' Care

Mr Broten: — Mr Speaker, the Premier has previously said in this House that health care workers should have no fear in speaking out about their concerns and about their ideas. The Premier said that health care workers should ". . . feel completely confident, completely comfortable and protected in bringing forward any information they have in the interests of patient safety and patient care." He said that health care workers do not have to worry about bringing their concerns forward to Health Region officials, to the government, or to the opposition. And he said health care workers don't have to worry when they speak up and write letters to the editor. Is that still the Premier's position?

The Speaker: — I recognise the Premier.

Hon. Mr Wall: — Mr Speaker, certainly it's my position. It's the position of the Minister of Health, both ministers involved in health care. It would be the position of the government. I would take it from the member's line of questioning that there may be an example where this commitment's not been honoured and, if that's the case, we want to hear the details, Mr. speaker.

The Speaker: — I recognise the Leader of the Opposition.

Mr Broten: — Mr Speaker, I know Peter was looking forward to the opportunity to sit with the Premier and convey the concerns that he and care aids have experienced. And Mr Speaker, I think it's important for the Premier to clearly state that no retribution would be received for the words that he expresses because Peter is incredibly concerned about the care of seniors. He talks about horribly inadequate staffing levels. He says, on paper, it's roughly one care aid for 23 residents during the night, but in reality, it's usually just one care aid for 28 residents. And for part of the night, Peter says, they have just one care aid for 32 residents with dementia. He talks about residents with dementia fighting with one another or punching and kicking staff, and he talks about a quality of care for our most vulnerable seniors that is far from adequate.

Does the Premier recognise that these types of staffing levels are not safe and do not provide the quality of care that seniors deserve and require?

The Speaker: — I recognise the Premier.

Hon. Mr Wall: — Thank you very much, Mr Speaker. The government has understood, since we had the honour of first being elected in 2007, that the staffing complement was not adequate in terms of, not just seniors' care in Saskatchewan, but also in terms of acute care and the number of doctors practising. And that's why adding to the complement of health care workers has been at the top of the list of priorities for this government, spanning two different ministers of Health, Mr Speaker. It's why there are 400-plus more doctors practising today. And we've completely overhauled the process for attracting foreign-trained doctors. We're training more here in the province.

It's why there are 2,600 more, more nurses of every designation working in Saskatchewan today than there were when member's opposite were the government, when they had a chance to do more than talk and actually undertake some action, Mr Speaker. It's also why this government, specific to the member's question, has increased the complement of long-term and integrated care front-line personnel by almost 800 since 2007.

Mr Speaker, we know there's more work to be done in seniors' care. That's why in a very, very tight budget we were able to allocate additional resources for seniors' care, some $10 million more on top of some of the emergent funding we've already provided, Mr Speaker. We know that more is needed to be done. But I can assure members of this House that as we have increased resources for seniors' care, increased the complement of care aides, LPNs [licensed practical nurse], and nurses providing that care, so too will we be working for continuous improvement in the future.

The Speaker: — I recognise the Leader of the Opposition.

Mr Broten: — Mr Speaker, in speaking with Peter, he's very clear that staffing levels and the conditions that he and other care aids are working under have gotten worse over the past years, Mr Speaker.

And this government admits that they don't know if the dollars are getting to the front lines, and that's backed up by the experience of those health care workers who are coming forward. It was the minister himself who said, "I do want to have some assurance from the deputy minister that those are indeed going to the front lines of long-term care, and so we're working to confirm that." Mr Speaker, they know where they've spent when it comes to lean consultants and those with stopwatches, Mr Speaker. But when you speak to those on the front lines, it's a very different reality.

My question goes back to an earlier question that I had to the Premier, Mr Speaker. I asked if Peter can be assured that he will face no retribution for speaking out today. Can the Premier confirm that?

The Speaker: — I recognise the Premier.

Hon. Mr Wall: — Mr Speaker, that was his very first question, this member's very first question. I provided that answer; that remains the position of the government.

And so it started.

And into hell, I walked.

I SMELLED A RAT – A POLITICAL RAT

A year prior I had injured myself. My latest x-ray and ultra-sound tests had shown that my injuries had not healed, but had become worse. I found it difficult to manipulate both my elbows when weight was applied. Therefore, when I returned to work on April 1, 2015, I was placed on light duty. I had been removed from night shift. The letter to the union said that my employer could not accommodate my needs on the night shift. Therefore, I had been placed on day shift. It was a shift I was totally unfamiliar with.

I would need to meet with management to determine what work I could do. I met a hostile management team walking down the office's hallway. They were in no mood to carry a conversation. My Director of Care gave me a few chores to do. I then received another chore from the director of physiotherapy.

The chores were simple but time-consuming. I was to correlate beds to rooms. Identify and mark each one. When done, I was to wash every chair in the auditorium. And then I was to do a hand-washing audit. But to start my day I was assigned to the older (south) unit. I was to help with breakfast chores and to assist in getting a few ambulatory people dressed.

As I worked, many staff congratulated me on stepping forward and blowing the whistle. Several told me that they wish they had the guts to do what I did.

Many of my friends on social media congratulated me. Many more wrote letters/cards of support. Although I didn't feel that elated, I did thank all for their unabashed support. I felt that all in the Long-Term Care community could relate to the problems that had been occurring at my work. And I truly believed that my work colleagues would see the rationale of my whistleblowing and search for change. How wrong I was. The knives of revenge began to appear. They would strike deep, and senselessly.

At about 2:00 pm on April 16, 2015, I received a telephone call from my DOC. She said that she had the ADOC and a union shop steward in her office listening to the call. I was told that I was not to report back for duty until further notice. I was also told that I had been suspended with pay pending the results of an investigation into accusations against me. When I asked what those allegations were, I was told to contact my union. And then she hung up.

It would be remarkably stupid of me not to know this was coming. However, what I didn't know was the amount of duplicity staff would use to get rid of me, now a confirmed troublemaker.

After allowing the information to sink in, I contacted the union. They had yet to receive the email containing the accusations. It would take two hours before I received it by email. Suffice it to say it was a nasty document full of half-truths and innuendos.

As luck would have it, both my wife and I kept the information to ourselves. Our family is very close, and confidences between us are common. However, this was a rare occasion when no one was told about the email and its contents. It was a wise decision: on April 20, 2015, I received an email from my contact in the NDP camp.

She had heard about my suspension and wondered what the union had to say about the issue. She then asked me to contact her via phone or email.

I didn't have the chance to call her. I was awash with television and newspaper reporters. They wanted to know who I thought leaked the information of my suspension to them. I was also told that at least one reporter had received an email from the Premier's Director of Communications, identifying more than one complaint against me. They wanted to know who I thought would have released my private and confidential information. I was honest; I didn't know.

There was speculation that the Premier and his cronies were out to ruin a whistleblower, me. I had heard from my brother-in-law. He had sent me information regarding whistleblowers. It was clear a scant few escaped the lambasting that followed their actions as an agent provocateur. But then they all believed in what they were doing. They all believed they had right on their side. And if God were real he would surely walk hand in hand with them.

The media speculated that the unprovoked attack against me was designed to control the situation, to remove any vestige of guilt from the government. It was decided, and much later, the government should have considered my complaints and ensured the public of their strong support for seniors. The Premier chose the wrong path..

The media smelled a rat.

I smelled a rat.

On April 21, 2015, I received an email from the NDP's aide de camp.

She said that she had seen the news coverage on CTV and in the newspaper and thought that I had given an excellent interview. What was interesting was that she mentioned that several people had phoned into the NDP office wondering why I was under attack. Apparently, several said that I was very professional at my job; they couldn't understand why I was coming under fire. I couldn't understand it either.

That same morning the following appeared in all major newspapers in Saskatchewan:

Seniors Care Aide worker suspended for speaking out about conditions: NDP (CTV Regina/Stoon, Global Regina, CBC, MJ Times, PAHerald, SP, LP)

And so the great fiasco, perpetrated in part by the government, was kicked up several notches.

The report identified an apparent connection between my coming forward, and whistleblowing, to my suspension and the government's promise that I would not be punished for whistleblowing. I had told the media that the leak of information did not come from me or anyone associated with me. I further advised them that I found it very unlikely that it would have originated from my union.

I strongly suggested that my suspension was due to my coming forward with embarrassing details of abuse. The article went on to say that at least one of the allegations was made after I spoke out. It was also made clear that my coworkers had made the complaints. But then Dustin Duncan, the Minister for Health, spoke out about the situation, stating that the information given to the media was "provided in a fairly limited fashion, on a background basis to reporters."

I firmly believed I had been suspended because of my coming forward about abuse of elders. An email to the media from the NDP supported me on that. The Minister of Health denied that allegation, stating that: "Health Regions wouldn't take disciplinary action against an employee for speaking out about the conditions in which they work." He then followed up with, "he wasn't sure whether the ministry asked for the information or if it was provided by the Health Region. It isn't a normal course of action for a Health Region to notify the government of a suspension." However, it became known that the information came from the Health Region. It was a blatant breach of my privacy.

The Deputy Leader of the NDP suggested that it was an attempt by the Premier and his staff to discredit me. The Health Region issued a statement saying it does not typically notify the provincial government when an employee is suspended. "Situations where we have notified the Ministry of Health in the past of HR related matters are circumstances where there was significant organisational impact like shifting of several positions or when there are matters of public concern," it said.

In a related article, a columnist painted an even gloomier picture. The headline read: 'Gov't unkind to health employee.' In the article, the columnist believed there were times when politicians deserved the bad reputation they sometimes received. The issue raised concerns that the allegations made against me by my colleagues demonstrated suspicious timing. The NDP were quick to point out that six of the eight allegations against me occurred after I spoke out.

The NDP then pointed out that the illicit emails to the media came from the Premier's Director of Communications. The Minister of Health, Dustin Duncan didn't think it strange that my information was released to the media. What he did find strange was that I asked that no repercussions be brought against me. He also didn't find it strange to learn that I had an eleven-year-long clean record, except one disciplinary action which had since been expunged. That was until I spoke out.

The next day, April 22, 2015, a meeting had been arranged between my employer, the Health Region Labour Relations, and myself. The nursing home would hold the meeting 11:00 am. As always, I arrived at the meeting on time. The offices were strangely quiet, eerie. It seemed cold, damp and uninviting. The CEO's office door was closed as was the ADOC's, two people whom I thought should have been at the meeting. The Director of Care's office was open, but she was not there.

For ten minutes, I walked the hallway looking at various paintings that school children had done. I rather like art, my daughter is a professional artist. But today the paintings were just a blur as I tried to focus on the issue at hand.

Suddenly the DOC appeared. She looked concerned. Had I not heard that the meeting had been cancelled? Normally when two people speak to one another, the distance between them is measured in inches. The distance between us was closer to ten feet. If I ever felt it was going to be an uphill battle (and I did, often) that moment would be the catalyst.

I returned home annoyed. I had prepared for this moment. I was ready, with documents in hand. My mind went into overdrive. I wondered if all had been resolved, swept under the carpet, covered up. Perhaps the Ministry of Health had become involved and ordered a stop to whatever my employer and the Health Region were planning.

When I got home, I settled myself and then phoned my Union. Why did you not tell me the meeting had been cancelled? I asked. It was an error. My rep was new and was busy coming up to speed on the difficult issues she was about to face. It was an oversight. An email should have been sent, she said. There were no confirmed dates for the meeting, I was told. She wasn't sure what my employer and the Health Region had in mind. I would have to wait for the email confirming dates and times.

On that same day I received another email from my NDP contact. We had been talking about the possibility of me filing a complaint with the Independent Office of the Privacy Commissioner (IOPC). She felt that Premier Brad Wall and the Minister of Health had gone too far when releasing my confidential information. She told me that she had talked to their legal team and they agreed I had a good case. She assisted me in my initial contact with the privacy commission by drawing up the following letter of introduction to my case:

Attention: Ron Kruzeniski, Q.C., Information and Privacy Commissioner Dear Mr Kruzeniski, Q.C. Private, confidential information related to the status of my employment has been disclosed by the Premier's Chief of Communications and Operations, Ms Kathy Young, to members of the Legislative Press Gallery and other media. Premier Brad Wall has admitted in the Legislative Assembly and to the media in a public interview that he personally obtained the confidential information from the Saskatoon Health Region and that he personally made the decision to leak that confidential information to members of the media.

As such, I am writing to lodge a formal complaint against the Premier and his Chief of Communications and Operations.In his media interview earlier today, the Premier said, "It's not a leak if we want to make sure that there's information out there." He said, "I think it's very important for the people of the province, and other health care workers to know that our promise was not broken." He said, "The legislation prescribes that some personal information can be provided if it is in the public interest and I think this is very much in the public interest."

When asked how he came to such a conclusion, he said, "I think it's in the public interest when I've made a promise to someone on the floor of the Legislature that they will not have any workplace repercussions from coming here and raising questions, that we keep the promise."

Premier Wall told reporters, "I think you'd have a stronger case simply to not trust us, take us at our word, if no information is provided. So we made that calculation that, if there's some general information, hopefully, the media and therefore the people and therefore health care workers will know we didn't take this decision because he came to the Legislature." He went on to say, "The conundrum for me and the government is, if we simply don't do anything or say, no, no, just trust us, it had nothing to do with him coming before the Legislature, I think that's less credible for health care workers watching, for the people watching, than if there's some general information provided."

When asked how his office became aware of my employment status, Premier Wall said, "I inquired. And apropos of Section 29 of the

Act, I want to know, I asked, we want to make sure that a promise that I made was not broken."

I respectfully submit that nothing in the Freedom of Information and Protection of Privacy Act says that the Premier or his staff are allowed to release private information of an individual citizen to protect the Premier's reputation or the reputation of his government. Nothing in the Act says that the Premier or his staff are allowed to release private information of an individual citizen to ensure that the public knows that the Premier has not broken a promise.

Nothing in the Act says that the Premier or his staff are allowed to release private information of an individual citizen to help the Premier and his government out of a "conundrum." And nothing in the Act says that the Premier or his staff are allowed to release private information of an individual citizen to present a "more credible" argument to those are paying attention.I am highly concerned that this intentional breach of my privacy by the most powerful person in our province is likely to have significant damaging and lasting effects on my reputation, and certainly on my future employment.

I also firmly believe that were Premier Wall and his office to get away with this significant breach of my privacy, it would set a dangerous precedent allowing politically motivated releases of information, allowing the Premier and his government to run roughshod over the fundamental privacy rights of individual citizens.

Thank you for your attention to this matter. I will fully cooperate with your office in this investigation. I can be reached at…(removed). Sincerely, Peter Bowden

And thus my foray into the legal aspects of politics began. The investigation by the Privacy Commission would take one line of my triple offensive. The other two would be equally challenging: one would lead down the path of accusations of abuse, and the other would be the allegations of impropriety against me. It would become a battle that would consume my wife and me for almost a year. Daily discussions on the same subject would cause depression and bring us very close to giving up the fight. But my birthright is English (I am Canadian and have lived in this wonderful country for forty years). As with the RCMP always gets their man, so the expression 'never put an Englishman's back against the wall' rang true. I would fight on and to the bitter end.

The release of my private and confidential information to the government would lead me to retain a lawyer for litigating against all three parties: my employer; the Health Region; and the Ministry of Health. The second would find me in a cloistered, vault-like room, challenging the Health Region investigator. The third would wind its way toward arbitration.

I received an email from my union rep. She said that we would be meeting at Avord Tower on the 8th Floor. Avord Tower is downtown Saskatoon and close to the South Saskatchewan river.

On April 24, 2015, and on the same day as the first of four meetings with the lead investigator, I received a response from privacy commissioner. I was intrigued. With many down days, this email lifted my spirits. I read each word with relish.

Thank you for bringing your concerns to our office's attention. Before I speak to your specific complaint, I would first like to provide you with an overview of the role of the Office of the Information and Privacy Commissioner (IPC). The IPC is an office of last resort with oversight of The Freedom of Information and Protection of Privacy Act (FOIP), The Local Authority Freedom of Information and Protection of Privacy Act (LA FOIP) and The Health Information Protection Act (HIPA). As an office of last resort, we typically do not consider a breach of privacy complaint until it has first been brought to the public body for an investigation. Once the internal investigation is completed, if the complainant is not satisfied with the outcome of the investigation he or she may then ask our office to investigate.

For the purposes of the complaint you have raised with our office, we must ensure that we have enough information surrounding the complaint in order to proceed.

In the email below you have stated:

"Private, confidential information related to the status of my employment has been disclosed by the Premier's Chief of Communications and Operations, Ms Kathy Young, to members of the Legislative Press Gallery and other media. Premier Brad Wall has admitted in the Legislative Assembly and to the media in a public interview that he personally obtained the confidential information from the Saskatoon Health Region and that he personally made the decision to leak that confidential information to members of the media. As such, I am writing to lodge a formal complaint against the Premier and his Chief of Communications and Operations."

Prior to considering proceeding with an investigation, please provide us with details pertaining to the following:

What private, confidential information related to the status of your employment was disclosed? In your email you make reference to "your employment status", but this does not inform us what information about your employment status was disclosed. When was this information disclosed?

Who was involved with the disclosure? For example, you note that Premier Wall personally obtained the confidential information from the Saskatoon Health Region.

Do you know who within the Saskatoon Health Region disclosed your personal information?

Did you at any time share these particular details with anyone outside of your employer? If so, what and when?

In addition to the above, if you have written material that supports that a breach may have occurred, please include that as an attachment.

We would like you to be aware that our office can only investigate matters for which we have jurisdiction. Government institutions are subject to The Freedom of Information and Protection of Privacy Act. Section 2(2)(b) of FOIP specifically excludes offices, such as the Office of the Premier, as being a government institution. Section 2(2)(b) states:

(2) "**Government institution**" does not include:

(b) the Legislative Assembly Service or offices of members of the Assembly or members of the Executive Council.

You have also stated that Premier Wall personally obtained this information from the (deleted) Health Region. The HR is subject to The Local Authority Freedom of Information and Protection of Privacy Act. Therefore, if you believe that the HR released your personal information to Premier Wall, they would need to have authority to do so under LA FOIP. As it appears that the HR may have been involved with this incident, you may want to consider initiating a privacy complaint directed to the HR and any other public body that you believe may have inappropriately shared your personal information.

To initiate a privacy complaint, detail your privacy concerns in writing and direct your complaint to the Privacy Officer for the public body. You will need to wait a reasonable amount of time for a response from the public body. For your information, the Privacy Contact for HR follows: (removed)

For further information and resources please visit our website at www.oipc.sk.ca.

Thank you, and if you have any questions, my contact information follows. (removed)

April 27, 2015, I answered the IPC email as best I could, with the invaluable assistance of my NDP contact.

To your questions:

What private, confidential information related to the status of your employment was disclosed? In your email you make reference to "your employment status", but this does not inform us what information about your employment status was disclosed.

The information that was released was done so by Kathy Young, the Chief of Operations and Communications, in a note to several reporters. It highlighted that I had faced discipline for 9 complaints and included details surrounding the allegations including examples in four cases. This issue is well highlighted in the articles below.

When was this information disclosed?

In an email sent to reporters on April 20th, 2015.

Who was involved with the disclosure? For example, you note that Premier Wall personally obtained the confidential information from the Saskatoon Health Region. Do you know who within the Saskatoon Health Region disclosed your personal information?

This remains a mystery to myself as well as to the media. As of Monday the 20th, Kathy Young had more information on my personal confidential HR file than I had been given. I was merely told on Thursday the 16th I was suspended with pay and not to come to work. I had no detail of the allegations until my meeting on Friday the 24th. The Health Region CEO claims there was "no detail" given to government officials yet Young's email included the number, category and examples of the supposed allegations against me.

Did you at any time share these particular details with anyone outside of your employer? If so, what and when?

I did not and could not have shared these details in advance of the privacy breach on April 20th. I had no details related to my file until after the memo came from the Premier's office. The fact that the Health Region, the Premier, his Director of Communications and members of the media had more information on my personal human resources file than I did is outrageous.

When it comes to the Privacy Commissioner's Jurisdiction, I think you do have jurisdiction to investigate. When I look at the Freedom of Information and Protection of Privacy Act, it says that the "head" of the government institution is "the member of the Executive Council responsible for the Administration of the agency." That's Premier Wall, and he should be held responsible for the release of my personal information. Even Premier Wall thinks that he is the "head" and that the Act applies to him because he keeps making reference to the "public interest" section of the Act to justify his actions.

I think it's really important for your office to examine all the facts of this matter, and I also think that you should interpret the Act so that Premier Wall is understood to be the "head" of Executive Council. He is continually defending his actions under section 29 as it relates to providing personal information in the public interest. He has said that the benefit to the wider public in knowing what is alleged against me outweighs any damage done. The premier rightly sees himself as subjected to these regulations and should be held to the standards of the Act.

To not consider the Premier, the head and fully investigate this breach of privacy sets a dangerous precedent for the handling of public citizen's information.

I am concurrently dealing with the Health Region as it relates to this issue, but I request that your office investigate these matters specifically as this breach of privacy has not only had incredibly damaging impacts to my reputation, employment and relationships, it has become of great interest to the Saskatchewan public at large.

The Premier had hidden behind the Privacy Act using section 29 to release my private information. This part of the Act stated that he might do so if it was in the public good. I questioned what good would be served for the public to know the complaints against me. Therefore, I used the Whistleblowers Act, believing I would be protected. I was wrong, dead wrong.

It is not necessary to read the following Whistleblower Bill, but it does make interesting reading. It also raises some very curious political issues.

BILL No. 609

An Act to provide protection, rights and remedies for certain employees (Assented to)

HER MAJESTY, by and with the advice and consent of the Legislative Assembly of Saskatchewan enacts as follows:

Short title

1 The Whistleblower Protection Act.

Interpretation

2 In this Act:

(a) **"employee"** means any individual who performs services for or under the control and direction of an employer that is a public agency or public institution for wages or other remuneration and includes applicants for employment, former employees or an authorised representative of an employee;

(b) **"public agency"** means any agency, board, bureau, commission, ministry, office or other branch of the public service of the Government of Saskatchewan and includes any Crown corporation or institution as the minister may designate;

(c) **"public institution"** means:

(i) a regional health authority or an affiliate, as defined in The Regional Health Services Act;

(ii) a university, college, institute, board of education or conseil scolaire, the conseil général or any other educational institution or body;

(iii) a municipality or other local governing body;

(iv) an institution or body that is subject to audit by the Provincial Auditor within the meaning of The Provincial Auditor Act;

(v) any other institution or body designated by the Lieutenant Governor in Council as a public institution for the purposes of this Act;

(d) **"reprisal"** includes threatened or actual discharge, suspension, reprimand, demotion, harassment, constructive dismissal, blacklisting, involuntary transfer, assignment or deployment or the refusal to hire an employee, or other adverse employment action taken against an employee with respect to the employee's terms and conditions of employment, or other actions which interfere with an employee's ability to engage in a protected activity as set out in section 3;

(e) **"supervisor"** means any individual with an employer's organisation who has the authority to direct and control the work performance of the affected employee or who has authority to take corrective action regarding the violation of any law, rule or regulation of which the employee complains.

WHISTLEBLOWER PROTECTION
Protected activity

3 No reprisal shall be taken against an employee of an employer that is a public agency or public institution because the employee does any of the following:

(a) discloses, threatens to disclose or is about to disclose to a supervisor, a public agency, public body, public institution or to an independent officer of the Assembly, an activity, policy or practice of the employer, a co-employee or another employer, that the employee reasonably believes is in violation of a law, an enactment, rule or regulation promulgated pursuant to law or an enactment;

(b) provides information to, or testifies before, any public agency, public body, public institution or the Assembly that is conducting an investigation, hearing or inquiry into any violation of law, or a rule or regulation promulgated pursuant to an enactment or law by the employer or another employer;

(c) discloses, threatens to disclose or is about to disclose to a supervisor or to a public agency, public body, public institution or to an independent officer of the Assembly an activity, policy or practice of the employer, a co-employee or another employer, that the employee reasonably believes is incompatible with a clear mandate of public policy concerning the public health, safety or welfare, or protection of the environment;

(d) discloses, threatens to disclose or is about to disclose to a supervisor, to a public agency, public body, public institution or to an independent officer of the Assembly any information regarding financial mismanagement of public money or other similar wrongdoing;

(e) assists or participates in a proceeding to enforce the provisions of this Act;

(f) objects to, opposes or refuses to participate in any activity, policy or practice which the employee reasonably believes:

(i) is in violation of a law, rule, enactment or regulation promulgated pursuant to law or an enactment;

(ii) is fraudulent or criminal;

(iii) is incompatible with a clear mandate of public policy concerning the public health, safety or welfare, or protection of the environment; or

(iv) involves financial mismanagement of public money or other similar wrongdoing.

Preservation of records

4 Notwithstanding any other enactment, any document, record or computer file that may be required for an investigation or disclosure pursuant to section 3 must be preserved.

Anonymity

5 The anonymity of any employee who provides information, testifies or makes a

disclosure pursuant to section 3 shall be maintained where circumstances warrant.

WHISTLEBLOWER PROTECTION

Forum

6 An aggrieved employee or former employee may, within one year, institute a civil action in a court of competent jurisdiction if a violation of any provision of this Act occurs.

Burden of proof

7(1) Subject to subsection (2), a violation of this Act has occurred only if the employee demonstrates, on the balance of probabilities, that any behaviour described in section 3 was a contributing factor in the reprisal alleged in the complaint by the employee.

(2) Relief may not be ordered under section 6 if the employer demonstrates by clear and convincing evidence that it would have taken the same unfavourable personnel action in the absence of the employee's behaviour.

Remedies

8(1) All remedies available in common law tort actions are available to an employee whose suit, claim or action brought pursuant to this Act is successful.

(2) A court may also, where appropriate, order any or all of the following:

(a) an injunction to restrain continued violation of this Act;

(b) the reinstatement of the employee to the same position held before the reprisal, or to an equivalent position;

(c) the reinstatement of full benefits and seniority rights;

(d) the compensation for lost wages, benefits and other remuneration.

Posting

9 Employees' protections and employers' obligations pursuant to this Act shall be conspicuously displayed and made available to employees of employers of public agencies and public institutions.

Existing rights not affected

10(1) The provisions of this Act are in addition to and not in substitution of or derogation of any rights or benefits that an employee may have pursuant to any collective agreement that governs that employee.

(2) Nothing in this Act shall be deemed to diminish the rights, privileges, or remedies of any employee under any other federal or provincial Act, law or regulation or under any collective bargaining agreement or employment contract.

(3) No employee may waive by way of a private contract any right set out in this Act, except as set out in section 11.

(4) No employee may be compelled to adjudicate his or her rights under this Act pursuant to a collective bargaining agreement or any other arbitration agreement.

Settlement

11(1) The rights afforded employees under this Act may not be waived or modified, except through a court-approved settlement agreement reached with the voluntary participation and consent of the employee and employer.

(2) An employer may not require an employee to waive, as a condition of settlement, his or her right to reasonably engage in conduct protected pursuant to section 3 of this Act.

Printed by the authority of the Speaker of the Legislative Assembly of Saskatchewan 2009

Prohibition

12 No employee shall bring or make any allegation knowing it to be frivolous or vexatious.

Crown bound

13 This Act binds the Crown.

Coming into force

14 This Act comes into force on assent.

This bill did not receive Royal Assent. It died on the order paper when the Legislature was prorogued in lieu of new elections. When the Saskatchewan Party came to power, the Bill never found its way to the House again. Both the government and the NDP must have thought there was little political merit in revisiting Bill 609. Employees stepping forward to lodge a complaint against healthcare had no protection except that from IPC. It seems callous that a simple bill like this would never see the light of day.

I had assumed Bill 609 would protect me. That I could come forward with my abuse complaints and still retain my employment. Did I ever get that wrong!

Politicians are supposed to be smart. They have a plethora of employees in their offices to guide them. They have access to solicitors and past laws to guide them through the maze of legal mumble jumble. The Office of the Premier is staffed to give sound, solid advice to the Premier and to ensure nothing is misspoken.

Through poor advice or against sound judgment, Brad Wall had slithered into a trap, a trap that became inescapable. He had inadvertently raised the issue of my suspension, calling it "discipline". He stated this in the House and drew the ire of Cam Broten who attacked him and his credibility as a protector of whistleblowers.

The trap? It was not possible for me to be disciplined. There had yet to be an investigation. The Premier had just told the public what the eventual outcome of the inquiry would be. Did he and his cronies know what the future held? Was this the thin end of the wedge? I certainly thought so as did the media, who had clung to every word the damaged Premier said.

Under pressure from the opposition and the media, Premier Brad Wall said in the Legislature that he would let the Privacy Commission do its work.

The media smelled a rat. Their respective mouths must have been salivating as they poured over computers and readied TV cameras. It was a good story, a true story. And yet, somewhere in the melee, the message was lost. Elderly people were suffering. It seemed to me the sensationalism of a whistleblower pitted against the Premier had overshadowed the message.

As much as the media smelled a rat, I also smelled it. But I looked at it from a different angle. I believed the allegations given me on April 24, 2015, were because of my whistleblowing. And reading those allegations fully, I became convinced my colleagues had conspired to condemn me. I couldn't help but wonder what role management performed in this sordid play.

And then there was the Health Region. Surely the Office of Labour Relations is staffed with intelligent people. They must have weighed the risks of getting involved. They certainly had all the documents to prove that I was right, that I spoke the truth, that my employer was short-staffed. Of course, they must have known short staffing leads to a lowering of the prescribed standards of care. Lowering of those standards leads to the neglect of residents. I had proof on my side. But then I didn't know it at the time. Eventually, I would go through the process of investigation and successfully litigate the government.

So, what happened to bring this conspiratorial judgment to the fore? Thoughtlessness, silliness and stupidity. The whole bloody mess could have been dealt with many months before my blowing the whistle. I would still be working as a Care Aide, and no one would be the wiser.

The Health Region could have contacted me after being informed of the infractions. They could have resolved the issues in short order.

The Ministry of Health could have sent it back to the Health Region and then to my employer. The Premier could have told his Director of Communications to do nothing with the information she had received.

Instead of doing nothing, each level in our health care system bungled. Each passed the buck. No one stood to take responsibility, to shut the matter down. When I returned to work on April 1, 2015, I fully expected to be dragged into the DOC's office, kicking and screaming. I anticipated being drawn over the coals and then sat down to discuss a resolution to the problem.

But then I was a whistleblower. I was in a different ball game on a different field. I had no idea the knives were being sharpened. There was no understanding the disgust I felt. I had spoken the truth and was now, like the proverbial lamb, being drawn to slaughter because of it. It was a warning to any other health care provider. Lest you want the same treatment, never complain, ever.

It was time to discover what a real whistleblower was.

THE LITTLE OLD LADY

She was a frail elderly lady, a lady with a sense of humour and a song in her heart. The severe curvature of her spine caused by osteoporosis gave her an all-too-familiar hump on her upper back. As she walked the hallways at night, she looked like Quasimodo.

Facts and Figures of osteoporosis

- Fractures from osteoporosis are more common than heart attack, stroke and breast cancer combined. Osteoporosis affects both men and women.
- Osteoporosis is often called the 'silent thief' because bone loss occurs without symptoms unless one has fractured.
- Osteoporosis can result in disfigurement, lowered self-esteem, reduction or loss of mobility, and decreased independence.
- Peak bone mass is achieved at an early age, age 16-20 in girls and age 20-25 in young men.
- The overall yearly cost to the Canadian healthcare system of treating osteoporosis and the fractures it causes was over $2.3 billion as of 2010. This cost includes acute care costs, outpatient care, prescription drugs and indirect costs. This cost would rise to $3.9 billion if a proportion of Canadians were assumed to be living in long-term care facilities because of osteoporosis. (The burden of illness of osteoporosis in Canada, Tarried et al., Osteoporosis International March 2012)
- Twenty-eight percent of women and 37% of men who suffer a hip fracture will die within the following year.
- Each hip fracture costs the system $21,285 in the 1st year after hospitalisation, and $44,156 if the patient is institutionalised (Long Term Care, author note).

- Osteoporotic hip fractures consume more hospital bed-days than stroke, diabetes, or heart attack.
- Fewer than 20% of fracture patients in Canada currently undergo diagnosis or adequate treatment for osteoporosis.
- A study recently reported that only 44% of people discharged from hospital for a hip fracture return home; of the rest, 10% go to another hospital, 27% go to rehabilitation care, and 17% go to long-term care facilities.
- One in three hip fracture patients re-fracture at one year and over 1 in 2 will suffer another fracture within five years
- (Osteoporosis Canada)

My resident also suffered from COPD (Chronic Obstructive Pulmonary Disease). I never knew the cause. The disease of the respiratory system includes chronic bronchitis and emphysema. As time went on her disease became worse. Breathing for her became more difficult. Whenever she awoke, usually around 1:00 am, I would go to her room. I would try to settle her back to bed. But it soon became a useless exercise. Finding her fully awake I would take her hand in hand to the dining room. She was a fast walker. I tried to slow her for the faster she walked, the more difficult it was for her to breathe.

She was truly a Canadian for she loved coffee and would drink three or four small cups while I sat with her. This was my favourite time of night. I was with those residents that were awake.

She was a very short, less than five feet tall. I imagined she would have stood over 5' 4" before osteoporosis stepped in to impede her height. And as small and frail as she was she had the energy of three women. She walked briskly, as though she was late for a bus. I kept on having to tell her to slow down the coffee pot was hot and it wasn't going anywhere.

As with most residents, when she first arrived she was anxious and restless. She was constantly walking out of her room and wandering the hallways. Each time she left her room the alarm would trigger on my pager warning me that she was wandering. Because she was ambulatory, the only alarm she did not have was a bed sensor.

Within an hour of her waking, other residents would begin to wander. Coffee or tea became the drinks of choice. The coffee, of course, was decaffeinated. At first, it was difficult for me to settle them, so I gave them toast or oatmeal. They ate voraciously. Within the hour most had returned to bed and slept well the remainder of the night. My frail little resident stayed awake refusing to go to her room.

Giving residents food at night and then settling them raised the spectre that they were perhaps hungry. Many of those awake were mostly large. Supper was at 5:00 pm with a light snack, usually a cookie, at 8:00 pm. I charted each incident and the amount of food eaten. As I look back on it, no one appeared concerned. It is a fact dementia residents wander at night. But it was how they settled after they ate a quality snack that should have drawn some response. Alas, it did not.

Perhaps they needed more food at suppertime. Perhaps they needed a larger snack before bed. The evidence was there. It was too obvious to ignore. But I'm afraid it was. As time went on residents wandered less and less. Dementia was taking its toll on simple freedom of movement.

As time wore on my little resident became increasingly agitated. Dementia was winning; she was rapidly deteriorating. Medication was the only route we could go to lessen her agitation. Often there is a reaction to an action. In this case, the side effects of psychotropic drugs were disagreeable to resident and staff alike. Once a bright, cheerful person, we would see in her a constant stupor. Simple commands were no longer understood. And she was in constant danger of falling. I was concerned for her wellbeing.

It left nurses and doctors in a conundrum. To give her medication to lower her agitation would, without a doubt, increase the risk of her falling. The real danger of fracturing bones was due to her osteoporosis. But she had to be stopped from fighting with other residents. Apparently, brawling with one resident, in particular, had become a common daily occurrence. The conundrum crossed all shifts; however, it was the night shift that had the greater challenges. When she was out and about during days and evenings, she spent them within sight of staff. There was five staff on day shift and four on evenings. When it came to nights we had one for up to four hours and two for the remainder of the shift.

Before her medication therapy, our little old lady could find her way back to her room after her night-time snack without bothering anyone. Times, however, had changed for now she endlessly wandered into other people's rooms. A multitude of alarms would trigger on my pager. Answering the alarms, I would find a plethora of doors open with their occupants awake. And no matter the numerous times I returned her to her room, I would not get back to the nursing station office before door alarms went off once again. My little old lady was back at it.

The insidious slide into dementia disease can be described as sloth-like. Small, seemingly insignificant events begin to build. My first clue that the slide had started in earnest was when my little old lady argued about going back to bed after her late-night snack. She demanded more coffee. I found it easier to offer a bribe. One more cup of coffee if she promised me she would return to bed afterwards. There was an agreement. However, due to the very limited memory of dementia residents, I had to sit with her and constantly remind her of our pact. At first, our pact remained sound, but, not long into the agreement, she decided that she would return to her room only after the fourth cup of coffee. She could still toilet herself. I was grateful for that.

She was always eager to dress herself, and did a fine job of it. Her clothes were always dark, blacks and greys. Many wore clothing of this drab colour combination. It seems as though any sense of colour had failed them during their later lives. I would always try and find some coloured clothing for her, especially on a Sunday. With fingers crossed I would search the used clothing boxes in each linen cupboard not only to find vibrant clothing but clothing of the right size.

The used clothing came from residents who had passed away. Families had little need of them. Therefore a grateful staff accepted all, even shoes and sneakers and the odd pair of slippers, although they tended to be well worn.

She liked to wear shoes, and we tried to accommodate her in every way we could. She did, however, have severe limitations when it came to cleanliness. She became increasingly dependent on my partner and me to get her ready for the day. It was yet another step in her rapid ageing. As time went on, we found that she began layering her clothes. To find her wearing several blouses and a couple of sweaters was not uncommon.

She was becoming confused. She began to put the clothing from her wardrobe and drawers onto her bed. At first, they were in the proper order. As time went on her clothing was just dumped on the bed in a haphazard way. Her sense of competence and understanding had left her for good. It was always a sad day for me when that realisation dawned.

When we did her peri-care, there was no fight but acceptance. Initially, when independence has been lost, many residents fight the change their loss of stature. It takes a little while for them to accept the adjustment in their lives.

Her breathing had become more difficult. Our little ladies blood oxygen saturation levels had reached a point where she required supplemental oxygen. This was supplied by way of a portable concentrator.

There is sufficient evidence to suggest those suffering from shortness of breath do not like anything over their faces. Even a nasal cannula can be sufficient to cause a false sense of alarm when trying to breathe. The little old resident would never keep her cannula in her nose. Within five minutes of me putting it in, I would find it on the floor. Up until the night she died, it would be an interminable battle of wills, a battle she would always win.

Oxygen delivered through a concentrator tends to dry nasal mucous membranes. It is not unusual to find people with a nasal cannula having nosebleeds. Because our resident wouldn't keep the cannula on, she didn't suffer from this malady. The concentrator comes equipped with a connector allowing a bottle of sterile water to moisturise the oxygen. This simple step makes breathing easier as the wearer is more likely to tolerate the oxygen. However, our resident was never afforded this relief, at least not until the end. The rules for the delivery of oxygen are quite clear. It would appear as though we were following them.

Oxygen delivered by nasal cannula at a rate of 4 Lpm (litres per minute) or less will *not* be routinely humidified for adult patients. All oxygen administered to paediatric patients should be humidified.

It was quite clear; the practice of humidified oxygen had been discontinued for routine application. I raised the issue with the nurse, but I did not receive a satisfactory answer. All I knew was that our resident refused to wear the nasal prongs for more than five minutes. I was never made aware of the above regulations and did not know them until I did research for this book. I wish I had known for her life might have been more tolerable.

Without supplemental oxygen, she was extremely anxious. She could not keep still, and she certainly could not sleep. The rare occasions when she did sleep with the oxygen running, she slept well. However, that was a very rare event. In her restlessness, she would take the tubing off and roll it in her bed sheets. Even though she may have been drowsy and needed sleep, we would have to strip her blankets to find the cannula. She would, of course, wake up. Almost certainly she would stay awake for the remainder of the shift.

It was not uncommon for me to find the oxygen tubing wrapped around the concentrator. After doing so, she would turn up the oxygen flow rate to the maximum 6lpm. And as frail as she was she had the strength to turn the volume dial until it jammed. She was becoming a danger to herself.

The protocol for a resident with her diagnosis was to raise the head of the bed to the semi-fowlers position (45 degrees). In this position, her ability to breathe became easier. She was still ambulatory and walked about at night with little effort until she ran short of breath.

Several studies show that using oxygen at home for more than 15 hours a day increases the quality of life and helps people live longer when they have severe COPD along with low blood oxygen levels. Oxygen therapies have good short and long term positive effects in people who have COPD. Using oxygen may also improve confusion and memory problems. It may improve impaired kidney function caused by low oxygen levels. (WebMd)

We would radio the nurse when the resident was short of breath. We were instructed to place the oxygen on the resident. In practice, it is the RN's responsibility to apply oxygen as this action an invasive procedure. But it was forfeited to Care Aide staff, thereby leaving the nurse to carry on with whatever she was doing. Not necessarily dangerous in its execution, but without knowledge of lung capacity and the required oxygen flow rate, damage

It must have been very difficult for day staff to keep an eye on our little lady. Her room was the farthest possible from the nursing station.

To alleviate the problem, the day nurse (our infamous LPN) arbitrarily transferred the resident to the family room. This room had no hook up for alarms. And as I was working on my own at night it was impossible to keep my eyes on her. Further, the room was in such a position I could not observe her without sitting in the room. To have her in that room at night seemed a silly idea.

When asked, the day nurse consistently repeated the LPN's excuse by stating that she and her staff needed to observe the resident and at all times. I argued, and strongly that the resident was still ambulatory. It would be better if she were returned to her room. The alarm system would be functioning, and we would have a warning of any movement. And although she was well aware of the limited staffing levels at night, her illogical rule won out. Management was drawn into the argument. Stupidity, it seems, shows no bounds for their answer was "You'll just have to make do. Days and evenings have to, so do you." Nights were damned by the ignorance of others. So as I did rounds, washed wheelchairs and stocked linen carts, without the ability to know what the little old lady was doing, I would find her doing what she did best: wander.

I had hit that proverbial brick wall. I was going nowhere. As usual, our nurse had joined forces with management. Although she understood the importance of room and resident alarms, I was damned by her inability to show courage in the face of absurdity. I was on my own. I had assured myself that my little old lady's health and security were my priority. I needed to know what she was doing at all times. No one, neither the RN nor management, understood or wanted to understand.

To break what I thought to be an impasse, I suggested that nights move the resident to her room and return her to the family room at the beginning of the day shift. That idea too was dashed as management raised the same silly answer as they had done previously.

My head hurt. I was beating it against a brick wall of stupidity, and I was getting nowhere. But then the resident was suffering as well. Her care was being compromised. Her basic needs could not be met unless I stayed with her. Then other resident's basic needs could not be met.

I came away believing day staff were by and large lazy. They didn't want to run to the resident's room several times during their shift. They certainly gave no thought to the night shift. They gave even less thought to the resident.

Was it abuse? I truly believe it was; of staff, that is. More could have been done to help us. A healthcare sitter could have been employed to watch over our resident. They are economical when compared to a Care Aide. But of course, there was insufficient money in the budget for such extravagant expenses.

For the next several months I would find the resident attempting to get out of bed. I would often find her crawling on the floor or sitting haphazardly in a dining room chair fighting for air. Unceremoniously she would pull the oxygen prongs from her nose, throw the tubing to the floor and then try to get somewhere, anywhere away from the family room. Her room had a window. This one had four blank walls. It was stark, depressing.

In her room, our little old lady had a bathroom. Because she could ambulate, I surmised she could have used it. In the family room, there was nothing. She had nowhere to go to relieve herself. I would often return from rounds or cleaning wheelchairs to find her sitting in the dining room with head down and having a difficult time breathing. She and her bedding were wet. I often found a pool of urine on the floor. She was trying to find a bathroom, her bathroom.

When she finally returned to her room, she stayed there. She was dying. She had lost the ability to walk, to talk. It was as if no one wanted her, to be with her. She was shut away from everybody and everything. This was the time she should have been in the family room.

But she was on her own. There was no family with her. Staff would have been nearby to comfort her and to attend to her needs. Alas, that was not the case. I was saddened to see such ignorance win over rationale. To allow my resident to suffer was, for me, a complete injustice. I made my point very clear during the investigation.

Indeed, her death marked the beginning of the end of my tenure in Long Term Care.

Excerpted from SHRA Residents Rights and Responsibilities.1. You have the right to be treated with consideration, respect and dignity.

6. You have the right to a safe environment.

With respect to understanding their rights, residents rely on their families and their care team to demonstrate increased vigilance in ensuring that their rights are respected.

11. With respect to residents who are unable to take responsibility for following guidelines, policies and procedures, again, families and the care team have an increased responsibility to act on behalf of the resident. For example, to ensure safety, rooms should be free of excessive clutter. A resident unable to follow this policy on his or her own would rely on families and the care team to work together to remove unnecessary items and keep the room tidy and free of hazards.

Safety is a responsibility of all members of the LTC (Long Term Care) community including the care team, residents, family members, visitors and volunteers. Residents and families are vital in the role of promoting safety and are included to the degree that they are able to prevent and report adverse events. The care team is trained to identify, reduce and manage risk. Everyone is encouraged to identify potential safety risks and report them to the appropriate person. Saskatoon Health Region and the management of Long Term Care homes follow up on reports and work to prevent the problems from recurring. (SHR resident's rights and responsibilities).

There is no doubt a good portion of the Residents Rights were not adhered too. The LPN and management clearly failed in their respective duties to this resident. It was indeed a sad time for me.

The end came for my resident in the morning after I left shift. Returning to her room, she was once again being watched over by the alarm system. Her rapid, jerky movements would trigger the bed alarm. I would find her sliding down the bed and off the sensor. At this stage, I would do nothing without my partner, and so I put out the call. Within ten minutes she joined me.

The resident's head had been raised the customary 45 degrees to aid her breathing. For the first time since being on oxygen (it had been nearly four months) it was humidified. And for the first time, she hadn't removed the nasal cannula. I could only surmise that the humidified oxygen was comforting. She was happy to keep it on. However, my little old lady was very agitated. Her arms and legs seemed to have a mind of their own. It was impossible to keep them still. And as we pulled her back up in bed, she was bound to slide down once again.

Her body writhed like a snake, and she was groaning lowly with each movement. She was in intense pain, of that both my partner, and I agreed.

While waiting for my co-worker, I spoke gently to her, trying to ease her anxiety. Whether she heard me I do not know. But it is recognised that the last sense to fail at death is hearing.

I talked about the past. The time she arrived on the unit. How she would consume coffee as if she hadn't had anything to drink for a week. When other ladies were up early in the morning, we would gather around a table and sing a few World War Two songs. How she kept her independence as long as she did. I talked about her friend and how they walked hand in hand along the corridor.

As I always did when someone was so close to death, I would say that the Great White Spirit of the North was waiting for her, to welcome her into his waiting arms. I would have said God, but as an atheist, I could not bring myself to lie to someone on the journey they were about to take.

Both my co-worker and I agreed she needed some medication to calm her and to reduce the pain. (My partner was from the Philippines. She was a well-seasoned RN. She had spent considerable time working as an RN in Saudi Arabia. She knew her skills). She had often worked nights in dementia and knew the residents well. We, therefore, both agreed that the rapid, jerky movements were very unusual and contrary to our resident's normal self.

I put a call into the nurse. While waiting for her arrival, we gently pulled the resident back up to the top of her bed. It was then I noticed a small bruise like mark on the side of one of her feet. It did not appear to be mottling, that tell-tale sign of impending death.

There are many **physical** signs of dying.

- Hands, feet and legs may feel cool or cold to the touch.
- Blood pressure gradually goes down, and heart rate gets faster but weaker.
- Fingers, earlobes, lips and nail beds may look bluish or light grey.
- A purplish or blotchy red-blue colouring on knees and/or feet (mottling) is a sign that death is very near.

Restlessness or agitation which may be a result of less oxygen to the brain, metabolic changes or physical pain. (Compassion and Support)

I checked her capillary refill by gently pressing on her large toenail. I squeezed the blood from under the bed of it. I watched her nail refill with blood. I timed its return. It was within five seconds, a more than acceptable time. I then checked for a pedal pulse. (The pedal pulse is on the top of the foot). As an EMT, I had been taught that if the pedal pulse could be palpated (felt), then there was a blood pressure of at least 90 systolic.

I found the pulse strong albeit arrhythmic, something expected at her later stages of life. I knew then the mark that I saw on her foot was indeed a bruise and not mottling.

The investigator was up to his old tricks. He was trying to suggest that Care Aides were not equipped with the knowledge to determine whether or not a resident was in the throes of death. Care Aides have been witnessing death ever since the term Care Aide (or aide) had been created. Indeed, it is fair to say personal Care Aides in any shape or form have been caring for aged, wounded and the sick since man first walked on this planet. But that little ditty was not good enough for the investigator. As I have stated prior, his charge, I am certain, was to bury me, the whistleblower. He contacted the SHRA Palliative Care Nurse Manager.

The investigator thought he saw a weakness in my story. Something perhaps he could pin on me. Something that I did that was undoubtedly wrong. He sent my charting of the resident's wound on her foot to the Palliative Care Nurse Manager for her assessment.

The nurse concluded that as I was not at liberty to analyse, the mark on the resident's foot was almost certainly misdiagnosed and that is was mottling. I stated quite clearly in my charting that I found a contusion like mark noted on outer aspect (side) of the right foot. Nowhere had I mentioned a confirmed diagnosis. I always made sure no diagnosis was ever made in any of my chartings. The charting in the Emergency Medical Technician programme was clear: never state a certainty. One must never speculate either. Describe what you see. A 'contusion-like mark' is not a diagnosis. However, to the investigator it was. To the Palliative Care Manager, it was. I stated quite clearly that I thought both were dimwits.

How, I thought, with the facts before her, could a palliative care nurse make such a mistake? I strongly suggested to my interrogator that this nurse was not capable of reading and understanding basic assessments. Further, I said that perhaps he/she should seek other employment where her type of skillset was not needed. In fact, I called her an idiot. I suggested to the investigator that if all managers were cut from the same cloth, then it is no wonder the healthcare system is in such a crisis. My interrogator was a manager; it was another dig at his pomposity.

I continued with my explanation of events. It took almost ten minutes for the RN to arrive. The time was not unusual. She witnessed the resident in an uncomfortable state. I explained that the resident's rapid movements and her whimpering were not normal. I stressed that she was in a lot of pain. I asked if anything could be done to help her get through to the end more comfortably. She said that she would check the med sheet to see if there was anything she could give the resident. When she returned (another ten minutes) she did so with a Tylenol suppository and, what I believed to be, Ativan, a drug to calm the resident. I was told that the drug was all the doctor had ordered. I was also told that Tylenol could only be given every four hours.

With the medication given I returned to my regular routine only to return to the resident a half hour later. Neither drug had made any difference. My resident was still writhing on the bed, and her moaning had become more frequent. It started to turn into a caterwaul. Tears of what I believed were pain drained freely from her eyes. The once-resilience of my resident had been broken by her lament. I knew she needed a stronger painkiller. Her journey toward paradise was fraught with the nightmare of pain and angst.

As I asked the nurse for something else to combat the pain. I was aware she would have to consult with the resident's physician. She would need a doctor's order to deliver a strong narcotic to calm her, to help with the pain and to carry her forward to her death. I radioed the nurse once more.

She came back to the resident's room. Again, I asked if there was anything we could do to help with the old lady's pain. Her answer became the catalyst for my complaint of abuse. She informed me that she would have to get a doctor's order to give her a narcotic. She would then need to start a PIC line (peripherally inserted central catheter, a small line inserted under the skin to provide medication). I was told that it was too late at night to call the doctor for orders. She then told me that the resident would have to wait until the day crew arrived. The LPN would then phone the doctor for the necessary order. It was four in the morning. I didn't understand why she didn't phone the doctor. It was her responsibility. I cursed her; I cursed the system and the whole rotten mess. My resident was in excruciating pain and was dying, and no one cared.

Needless to say, I was shocked. A nurse not stepping up to the plate to do her duty? To let a resident suffer when that suffering could be reduced, and dramatically? Whose very training was a firm promise to aid the suffering?

Kindness and empathy are essential. Patient's health and comfort will be the nurses first thought and tact. Understanding will often effect without difficulty what might otherwise distress and fret the patient.

The nurse must carry out all doctors' orders faithfully. Should she fail, she must immediately acknowledge her mistake. (British Red Cross Nursing Manual number 2)

Was the RN worried about phoning a doctor that time in the morning? Could she justify leaving a resident in extreme pain? Did she have the mettle to do her job properly?

Annoyed, speechless, I held onto my resident's hand as the nurse turned and left the room. My co-worker was equally shocked, silently staring at the hurt that writhed on the bed. I looked at my partner, and a million silent words flowed between us. I believe we both understood that our resident would suffer in pain through to the end. I just hoped that that end would come quickly.

The shift ended. I walked past the resident's room on my way out to the parking lot. Her writhing had been reduced to twitching. I knew the end was close. I had already said my goodbyes, so I kept on walking.

When I returned that night, I was told that she had died at eight-thirty in the morning. The LPN had checked her at seven-thirty. She stated in her report that the resident was still and appeared comfortable. It was the day staff that had found the resident deceased, or so one Care Aide informed me. However, according to the resident's chart, the LPN went to give her a Tylenol suppository at nine-thirty only to find the resident deceased.

During the investigation, the case was discussed and all the above mentioned. I was informed that my version of events didn't match what the night nurse had charted. I already knew that a few reports by this nurse had been falsified, after all, I had witnessed them. Therefore, I was not overly concerned. However, it appeared as though my partner had sided with the RN for the investigator had stuck to the RN's version of events never once mentioning my partner's role. I told him that my charting was correct and I would not stray from it.

And then he dropped a mini-bombshell. The facility carried PIC lines and sufficient opiate to reduce pain. The investigator told me that the RN had the ability to insert the PIC line and start the drug therapy so badly needed. And this could be done **without** doctors' orders. I scratched my head and wondered aloud why the procedure wasn't done. Was it sheer laziness, ignorance or perhaps it's just that she didn't care? I wish I knew…

The investigator wasn't there to answer my questions. I was there to answer his. That had been clearly stated. It appeared as though he was looking more at the professional organisation of registered nurses and their training rather than the very person who was there and in control throughout that fateful night. I had a deep-held feeling I was being blamed for bringing what he deemed wrongful information forward, to attempt to discredit the nursing staff.

My thoughts ran deep, and I slowed down. My speech stopped as I thought back to the reams of documents I had been allowed to see. I knew I had to discredit one of the nurses. I knew I had to put her in a situation where her charting was in doubt. My thoughts tore through the hours of testimony.

Then it struck. A home run, sort of.

A staff member had told me that the resident had died at eight-thirty that morning. I had no reason to disbelieve her. The infamous LPN had charted that the resident had died at nine-thirty. But then she gave a written submission to the investigator stating that the resident had died at ten-thirty. I threw my hands up asking loudly at what time did the resident die? He looked at me strangely. "The chart said, nine-thirty."

I told him that a responsible Care Aide informed me the resident died at eight-thirty. The LPN put the death at nine-thirty and yet in a brief to my interrogation she stated that the resident died at ten-thirty.

The interrogators his face turning slightly crimson, he tore back through the reams of evidence he had shown me. It took a few minutes, but he eventually found the damning brief the LPN had given. Sure enough, my version held out. No one knew at what time she died that morning. It was certain the LPN didn't. It was a small victory, a victory I would enjoy for a long, long time.

I tried to offer what I thought was a reasonable explanation. The LPN didn't know when the resident passed away because she was never there at the resident's bedside when she was alive, as suggested in her charting. I insinuated that the resident died at eight-thirty, as the Care Aides had told me, and that the LPN never looked at the old lady. I even suggested that the LPN fabricated her chart notes entering as she did that she had checked on the resident at seven-thirty. If she checked the resident at seven-thirty, she should have sought doctors' orders for the opiate. The night nurse would have instructed the LPN to do so. This is what she told us she would do earlier on that morning.

The LPN did not have the right to superimpose her innate personal knowledge on a resident's welfare over that of a Registered Nurse. However, this LPN was well-known for ignoring the night nurse's requests. Officially the RN was her superior. However, it would appear as though this indeed happened.

Further, the resident, I believe, died at eight-thirty. Because of charting the death long after it happened, the LPN simply got the time of death wrong. I further suggested that at no time was the doctor called for an order for pain medication because, by the time the LPN arrived, the resident was already dead.

I was strong to denounce both the Night Nurse and Licensed Practical Nurse. They had a combined attitude that made them superior to anyone else. The doctor will converse with them about residents and their state of health. The Care Aides, who have intimate knowledge of residents, are, by and large, ignored. I have witnessed it time and time again. And I have often found it detrimental to good care.

We all strive to deliver a standard of care with the resident as our seminal focus. Sometimes, many times, the resident is the last person on the focal plane.

Was the LPN irresponsible in her duty? Was the RN derelict in her duty? Did anyone listen to the Care Aides? Could the resident's pain have been reduced to allow her a more comfortable death? Had the charting of both nurses been corrupted to save them from disciplinary action? Whatever the case, the abuse of this resident was never raised again. And as I do not have access to my allegations of abuse report, I do not know what conclusions have been made.

Four people know the truth. Myself, my partner, the day LPN and the duty night RN.

The truth will eventually be told, and I shall be set free.

THE FACTS MA'AM, JUST THE FACTS

It is clear health care facilities have faced and will continue to face chronic problems with dilapidated and crumbling facilities.

Cam Broten discovered that a 2014 report pegged the repair bill for all health facilities in Saskatchewan at 2.2 billion dollars. The backlog was set at 935 million dollars in the Saskatoon Health Region. It would not be an understatement to suggest that healthcare in Saskatchewan is facing serious issues. The Premier, Brad Wall, stops at nothing to wrap his arms around immigrants to Saskatchewan, whether they be Canadian or refugees. He can bask in the sunlight of the present and hide in the clouds of the past. As he pours money into the dreams of our new neighbours, the old nightmare of a crumbling healthcare infrastructure falls further into disrepair.

These thousands of new Saskatchewanites will push the boundaries of sustainable healthcare by their very presence. Already, emergency departments in hospitals are swollen to maximum capacity. It is not uncommon to wait for six, seven, or even eight hours to see an emergency physician. And as much as the government says they are reducing the wait times, I waited almost fourteen hours before I saw an emergency physician. I then spent another fourteen hours before I was admitted. And my physician had made special arrangements to get me into the Emergency Department. Unfortunately, my case is not unusual. As I sat in that Emergency Department, which was engorged with the sick and injured, I discovered that many more were in the same predicament as me.

It's just a matter of time before the entire system collapses under the strain of underfunding.

Governments don't apologise. They make excuses. They point fingers. They don't care what damage they do or who they hurt as long as they come out of it whisker clean. Once elected they work hard to be elected once again. The problem is their constituents do not know the truth, only what they are told. They have built a brick wall between the constituent and themselves. In this book, I hope I have exposed how damning those who sit in ivory towers can be to their voters. Of course, it won't collapse. No government in their right mind would ever allow such a calamity. What, therefore, is the alternative? The priority for any government is to understand the problems facing healthcare. It is not good enough to say that in the last budget we gave seniors' care an extra 12 million dollars, and as a government, we are proud of that. It is good enough only when governments understand the depth of the problems and face up to them. Perhaps, in this case, the Premier should have said: "We have given 12 million dollars to seniors' care. We know it is insufficient. And we apologise." However, such astute language from a politician will never happen.

We are beginning to understand that the Saskatchewan government is short of revenue. During the good times, when revenue poured in like oil bursting from the ground, our government went on a spending spree. Unlike ordinary people, they didn't seem to care to save for a rainy day. In Saskatchewan when it rains it pours. And when the crunch came, and money was needed to bolster healthcare, the kitty was dry.

How then do we raise revenue to pay for new hospitals and Long Term Care Facilities? We could sit on the fence and wait for world oil to head back to 100+ dollars a barrel. But at the current price of 40 dollars a barrel and world inventories bulging, it's fair to say that could be a long, long time. Of course, the only other sure way of raising funds is through taxation and cuts. These are the obvious routes. Taxes have many avenues to squeeze us. Personal tax, gas tax, goods and services tax, airport tax, taxes on tires, bottles, clothing. It never ends. And of course, those that sin are true patriots of the government grasp. Every package of cigarettes or every bottle of alcohol becomes the target.

Building new facilities with new tax money would help go a long way to relieving the pressure on the healthcare system. But with all these new people entering the province more hospital beds will be required. More hospital beds require more staff. More staff means more training facilities. It is a conundrum that seems to have parked itself within our healthcare system.

It takes approximately four to six years to train a Registered Nurse, two to three years for a Licensed Practical Nurse, and nine months for a Continuing Care Aide. If supply can outrun attrition, then mathematically we could be ready. But now it appears retirees are outrunning the new influx of staff. There is, of course, an easy solution. Retain employees from outside of the country. That presents certain problems most of which are language and skills based.

There is apparently no sign of major expenditure on new construction. Money seems to be flowing for infrastructure. A new flow-through traffic system in Saskatoon recently opened. Two more bridges and a major road link are already under way. Regina is getting a multi-billion-dollar bypass. But the elected officials of both cities appear to shrink away from healthcare problems by pointing their elected finger at the provincial government, screaming: "It's their job!" And the provincial government likewise points their finger to Ottawa. Ottawa says it has no money. Honestly! There doesn't appear to be any hope.

It has become apparent to healthcare workers that the system has become management heavy. Each department in each facility appears to have a department head. Then, of course, each department head has their junior, someone who has made the grade but has upset someone along the way. Each, of course, needs a string of clerical staff, etc. It has become a bureaucratic nightmare. One only needs to look at the plethora of useless memos fired in all directions to understand the ridiculousness of it all.

Management, with their base salary, bonuses, performance bonuses, expense accounts, etc. drain away valuable resources while capital needed at the patient/resident level becomes ever more scarce. Perhaps it's time we asked management: "What do you do? Are you an important part of the everyday delivery of healthcare? Can we live without your skills? Or, can we amalgamate your skills with another?" Perhaps amalgamate several management positions. Reduce waste, reduce staff, reduce expenditures. Divert savings to where it is needed the most, the patient/resident bedside.

Perhaps we should be like private industry and give bonuses to those that show a focussed regard for their office. Those that save budgetary dollars reap the rewards of bonuses.

One does not have to look far to find waste and mismanagement. Except for minor additions and the elimination of one quote, the March 19, 2014, Long-Term Quality Assessment Report for the nursing home where I worked was the same as the June 10, 2013, report.

In the 2013 CEO Tours report, Sandra Blevins, Donna Bleakney and Lori Hinz were the three that represented the Regional Health Authority where I worked. It was those three CEO's that identified problems within the facility. Shortage of staffing at all levels was identified as chronic. In the 2014 CEO Tours Report both Donna Bleakney and Lori Hinz were once again assessing the same facility. And once again they identified short staffing as a chronic problem. There is little wonder why both reports look virtually identical. The question is, of course, were the women ever taken to task over the seeming paste and copy reports?

Staffing levels never did increase from 2013, leastwise not in dementia, and not on the night shift. Therefore, I would strongly suggest these CEO's performance, while perhaps credible, did little, if anything, to alleviate any of the identified problems. What it did do, however, was to show, from the investigator's point of view and presumably the Health Region's, that the resident council was not worth any weight when it came to complaints. It is indeed a sordid account of how those that sit on the council are treated by those hidden faces in ivory towers.

It is not good enough for the Minister of Health to stand in the Legislature and beat his chest while he attempts to stand guard for residents. It is only good enough when he stands tall in the Legislature and promises to right the wrongs. If those two CEO Tours Assessment Reports about my employer are indicative of other failings, then it's time we cleaned house.

I don't know what happened to those two women. Management has a funny way of circling the waggons around injured colleagues.

ABUSE, HOW DO WE KNOW?

Canada defines elder abuse as "any action by someone in a relationship of trust that results in harm or distress to an older person. Neglect is a lack of action by that person in a relationship of trust with the same result."

Canada is also a signatory to the United Nations definition of abuse.

There has never been a major academic study of institutional elder abuse prevalence in Canada. In the 1990's, the College of Nurses of Ontario conducted a survey of nursing staff and found that:

- 20% reported witnessing abuse of residents in long-term care settings
- 31% reported witnessing rough handling of patients/residents
- 28% reported witnessing workers yelling and swearing at patients/residents
- 28% reported witnessing embarrassing comments being said to patients/residents
- 10% reported witnessing other staff hitting or shoving patients/residents

In 2013, television documentarists W5 (CTV News), over the course of a one-year investigation, uncovered at least 1,500 cases of staff-to-resident abuse and neglect in nursing homes across Canada. It is believed that that number is much higher. But as we have seen, under-reporting is prevalent in health care facilities due to residents being frightened to come forward.

The W5 reporter, Sandie Rinaldo, asked three questions:

In the past year, have you witnessed staff-to-resident abuse (verbal, physical, emotional, sexual, financial) in the nursing home where you work?

To whom did you first report the incident?

Is the staff member who you witnessed abusing a resident still employed at the nursing home where you work?

There were 677 responses. It appears that many incidents go unreported.

38% reported having witnessed one of their colleagues abusing a resident

Only 51% said they reported abuse they had witnessed to a manager or administrator

More than 80% said that the staff member they had seen abusing a resident was still employed at the facility

Province or Territory Reported Incidents of abuse.
- Newfoundland and Labrador 3
- Prince Edward Island 0
- New Brunswick 10
- Nova Scotia 36
- Ontario 1,111
- Manitoba 59
- Saskatchewan 30
- Alberta 113
- British Columbia 138
- Northwest Territories 1
- Nunavut 1
- Yukon 0
- Total 1,502

Lynn McDonald of the University of Toronto's Institute for Life Course and Aging told Sandie Rinaldo: "There is a management issue of secrecy. There's no encouragement for anybody to report anything or do anything because they'll just get in trouble as these people know." (courtesy CTV News)

Abuse statistics for our neighbours to the south are equally horrific. In the United States, nineteen states reported substantiated mistreatment of the elderly, which included:

- Self-neglect (37.2%)
- Caregiver neglect (20.4%)
- Financial exploitation (14.7%)
- Emotional/psychological/verbal abuse (14.8%)
- Physical abuse (10.7%)
- Sexual abuse (1.0%)
- Other (1.2%)

Is there an answer? Can we see our way clear to resolving the situation? I believe we must bring all Continuing Care Aides into a professional fold. We must establish a professional organisation where education standards can be enacted and adhered to.

We must institute a governing body that licenses Care Aides. Equally, that same governing body should carry the burden of elder safety by removing licensees should a guilty infraction occur.

The governing body should maintain professional and ongoing training modules with consequences should they not be adhered to.

The governing body should consult with provincial Health Care departments to determine legal requirements for Care Aides.

The provincial government should set in place laws that govern Care Aides.

The provincial government should set in place a Standard of Care not only for those in Long Term Care facilities but also within the Department of Health, be they hospitals, Long Term Care facilities, private care homes and even elders in their home.

There must be an education program that begins at Kindergarten and continues through high school, teaching the virtues of elderly people.

We must all learn the doctrines of humanity, to treat one another as we would expect to be treated. It is not good enough to say: "He has dementia, he'll forget all about in a few minutes." It is only good enough to say: He's one of us, lived his life and deserves the best care we can give.

That's the big picture. But what about the smaller picture? The things that occurred where I worked and in particular the dementia unit and at night? Should I go as far as to exert blame?

Blame is simple. It is self-serving. It absolves and redirects. It is all encompassing. But it is not multi-directional. The finger of blame points one way and one way only. And that is up. That finger of blame continues until it finds the culprit. I will point that finger of blame even though it is self-evident throughout the text. The questions we must ask are: "Why did it happen? Why was it not stopped? And why, after such an exhaustive proving investigation, does it still continue unabated?"

In nursing, there is a command structure not dissimilar to the military. Complaints travel upwards. Commands travel downward. Directives travel in all directions.

The command structure in healthcare from bottom up is a little complicated. Thus, I'll review my employer's command structure, from the top down: The Health Region; The board of directors; Chief Executive Officer; all department heads; supervisors; us poor mortals, CCA's, housekeeping, laundry, dietary, etc. Without question, every complaint travels from bottom up.

Usually, a complaint from a Care Aide would travel to the LPN. From there to the duty nurse. And then upward. On night shift we did not have that first step. In dementia, we reported directly to the RN. I assumed that if a resolution could not be found then the complaint would take the next logical step and that would be to management.

Almost all information from night shift to management went via email. It would always flow through the nurse's email account.

Although each staff member had an active email account, I never used it to contact management. Any email received by the RN concerning care was dictated to staff. We were never allowed to read it.

As all information travelled to and from the nurse, trust became an important factor. I believed that all my complaints were reaching management. I was using the correct procedure. And although I was receiving no direct reply, a few of my complaints were obviously on the mark. But by the middle of 2014, things began to change, and without obvious reason.

The night shift RN is management in absentia. It is her responsibility to ensure the shift runs smoothly. She ensures all residents and staff under her command are safe. She is also the purveyor of justice. If she is unable to handle the situation, then management become the judge advocate.

The RN had chosen inaction on several occasions. My reports of potential skin breakdown, with photographs to back up those statements, were silenced. My horror at an LPN giving suppositories late in the evening likewise fluttered in the breeze. The statements of possible abuse were similarly ignored.

I am a conspiracy theorist. I believe collusion among staff brought about my downfall. I find it difficult to accept that management would deliberately withhold damning evidence against me and not allow me to speak in my defence. Not only that but somewhere along the line of probable conspirators, someone leaked my private and personal information to the Premier's office. The Premier's Communication Director then leaked it to the media. It is hard to believe that this course of events was nothing but a conspiracy. My employer, the Health Region, Saskatchewan Health and the Premier's office all knew, or should have known, what they were doing.

That this should never have happened is clear. Management should have been aware of the Health District policies and the protection of people like me who speak out. Obviously, they did not, or they were trying to terminate a Care Aide who was very vocal in advocating for his residents.

POLICIES & PROCEDURES

Number: 7311-10-003

Title: SPEAKING-UP - PROTECTION OF PERSONS REPORTING WRONGDOING

4.2 All staff and stakeholders

4.2.1 Promote a positive and ethical work environment.

4.2.2 Respect and operate within the bounds of internal controls and exercise diligence in detecting wrongdoing.

4.2.3 Report witnessed and suspected incidents of wrongdoing to their supervisor/manager. Anyone reporting a potential wrongdoing in good faith will not be penalised or reprimanded.

4.2.4 Do not discuss suspected incidents of wrongdoing with anyone inside or outside of SHR other than those who have a legitimate need to know such results in order to perform their duties and responsibilities.

4.2.5 Actively participate in investigations of wrongdoing.

4.2.6 Hold all suspected wrongdoing information received in the strictest confidence.

4.3 Directors/Managers/Supervisors

4.3.1 Review all reports received of suspected wrongdoings and forwards the alleged incident to the appropriate department (e.g. Risk, Privacy and Compliance, OH&S, Security, Labour Relations).

4.3.2 Share information only on a legitimate need to know basis, with senior leadership, the Authority, Audit and Finance Committee, and/or law enforcement agencies.

4.3.3 Conduct process reviews, as directed, that surround the disposition of each incident and to make process improvements that will assist in the detection and deterrence of similar events within their respective departments.

Whenever I start to point the finger of blame, I look at myself first. Did I do something wrong when I started out with my tales of abuse? According to the above policy, that is a resounding yes. I had clearly violated subsections 4.2.4, 4.2.6 and 4.3.2. But then I did adhere to the remainder of the policy namely subsection's 4.2.1, 4.2.3, 4.2.5, 4.2.6, and 4.3.1. What remains interesting is that until I started research for this book, I didn't know such a policy existed.

What did management fail to do? 4.3.1, which is a little ditty and 4.3.3, my interpretation of which is as follows:

Review all reports received of suspected wrongdoings and forwards the alleged incident to the appropriate department (e.g. Risk, Privacy and Compliance, OH&S, Security, Labour Relations).

I don't believe this was ever done, not until they were forced to by my coming forward the way I did, blowing the whistle. They had been told countless times that residents were not being treated properly. The word abuse was used in discussion with management on March 26, 2015, and yet they did nothing. They, I believe, decided to sit and wait for their conspiracy forces to gather sufficient blind evidence to force me out before the truth was ever established. It smacked of a cover-up.

As for 4.3.3? Well, that one was left to the investigator. He made a real hash of it by suggesting nothing untoward had happened. Not only that, but he also raised the spectre of solicitation, something that he is not allowed to do. He seems to have overstepped his mark to find favour with the executives of the Regional Health Care Board.

What surprised me the most about the inquiry? My colleagues. The truths we identified as we worked together on residents, discussing the very reason for my label of abuse, became a non-issue. The nurse who witnessed the very abuse I was concerned about turning a blind eye. The LPN who gave those suppositories to those residents late in the evening, showing absolutely no care or empathy to her residents. The investigator whose investigation was nothing more than a very expensive witch-hunt.

Had management taken steps to listen closely to my message then resident's lives would have been better. Their treatment at night would have dramatically improved. But the fact is no one cared. Neither the DOC nor her counterpart the ADOC ever, to my knowledge, stepped into the workplace to discover for themselves what was happening at night. The CEO likewise turned away from the problem. Each turned a blind eye, closed their ears and kept quiet.

Then, of course, there are the politicians. The crème de la crème of our esteemed society. Every four years or so we lend them our ultimate trust by voting for them. We expect a lot in return for our X on a piece of paper. But our politicians let me down and let down the very residents who were being abused. Had they stepped up to the plate, sought to rationalise what I was saying and sought a solution, you would not be reading this book.

Instead, political hay was made on one side of the Legislature while the other side decided to destroy the whistleblower. Both sides spoke what they wanted to be the truth. Trouble was only one side knew that truth. And for many days they delighted themselves in attacking one another's credibility. The problem was that no one visited the facility where I worked. Not one politician saw for themselves what the real situation was. They were far too busy in the daily media scrum, verbally battling one another. They were far too busy to worry about such minor trifles as our province's old people. And perhaps that is the problem with our politicians, all talk, no action.

It is very upsetting. Politicians are well remunerated, but for what? Being there; observing them; talking to them; I was left with the distinct impression they needed to stand in front of one another, like a bunch of ne'er-do-wells, beating their collective chests all the while shouting their mistruths hoping their political difficulties fade into the collective memories of a far off election. I would not call them liars; orators of deception is more of a correct term. Whatever the case, standing and arguing with one another (and in the public domain) did nothing to relieve the situation. And all the while the shouting was going on, Saskatchewan Health was slowly sinking into the abyss.

I did what I thought was right. Many healthcare professionals thanked me for coming forward, for bringing attention to something that had been left unchecked for far too long. And as I came out of the inquiry, a surfeit of very offensive testaments written by my colleagues was recited to me. It became a new low. Relationships honed over four years were sent to the waste basket of history, and I must live the rest of my life with those repulsive accounts of my person.

I also received a severe drubbing from the Right Honourable Premier of Saskatchewan, Brad Wall. It was unfair, unjust and irresponsible. And although I received written apologies from both Saskatchewan Health and the Health Region, and a verbal apology from the government by the Premier, I have as yet to receive any apology from my employer. As I expressed to my union, my employer must think themselves better than our government.

Not long after the investigation started I was asked by a reporter, would I do it again? Would I blow the whistle on abuse? It took no thought when I answered, "No!" Understanding the personal agony my wife and I were going through, the answer was obvious. Then reason flexed its muscle. "Yes, I would," I said, truth pushing past my lips. "How could I keep silent when people are suffering needlessly?"

I am a humanist. I was and am a strong advocate for my dementia residents. I believe in what I did. I became the first healthcare professional to come forward, to be a whistleblower. Of that, I am unabashedly proud.

THE NUMBERS

Saskatoon City Hospital was opened to the public in the fall of 1993. In 1991 the local census pegged the population of Saskatoon at 186,058. In 2014 the city census measured the population at approximately 253,000. It is estimated that by 2025 the population of Saskatoon will have reached 350,000, with a strong suggestion of a population of a million people within fifty years.

From the 2006 to 2011 censuses, those over the age of sixty-five grew by 12.8%, with males at 10.7% and women at 14.7%. Are we, therefore, prepared to look after the inevitable influx of the aged and infirm into Long Term Care homes?

The number of people living in rural Saskatchewan has grown dramatically. The catchment area for all three Saskatoon hospitals has grown exponentially, creating a bottleneck for the sick and injured. Since Saskatoon Hospital came online in 1993, we have seen a growth of nearly 100,000 people. It is no wonder people are complaining about line-ups at the emergency departments.

The fix seems simple. Build more hospitals. Unfortunately, that will not address the problem. Buildings themselves do not cure people. It takes nurses and doctors and management to fill the void. Unfortunately, there are not enough doctors to carry the load. Trying to find a doctor accepting new patients in Saskatoon is an all but impossible task. I would suspect a similar problem would exist in a hospital environment.

And then there are those that work in and run our hospitals and nursing homes, including (but certainly not limited to): Housekeeping, Laundry, Dietary, Maintenance, Continuing Care Aides, Licensed Practical Nurses, Registered Nurses and the relative newcomer, Practical Registered Nurses.

All this, of course, takes money, and lots of it. The Saskatoon Health Region's health budget for 2014-2015 was 1.156 billion dollars, which equated to 32 million dollars a day.

The following wages are based on that particular job title having reached the highest wage step, actively employed full-time. It does not include overtime, weekend bonus or shift premiums. It is based on 1920 hours of work and paid holidays/year and is current as of November 2015, wages. All numbers are approximate and are within a margin of error of +/- 3%:

Continuing Care Aide $44,160

Licensed Practical Nurse $67,200

Registered Nurse $86,400

Practical Registered Nurse $109,440.

RN's working overtime night shift will earn approximately $90.00/hour. An LPN, $52.5; a CCA will earn $34.5.

It has been known that a Registered Nurse in Saskatchewan had earned more than $164,000 in one year. This high income was derived from overtime, something that haunts health regions each day. The cost of short staffing translates into overtime. Not only does this affect the cost of budgetary restraints but it has the potential of putting lives of residents and patients at risk. It is indeed unsettling.

Science has worked hard to keep our population healthy, to avoid those maladies that would put the aged in Long Term Care homes. Treatment for strokes is dramatically improving. The recognition that speed to a hospital is vital to a more successful outcome is now common knowledge.

The heart attack survival rate is increasing; it is becoming less debilitating. Great strides are being made into research on Multiple Sclerosis. However, we cannot remove the accident that leaves someone with a fractured spine and therefore quadriplegic.

Self-help groups such as Al-A-Non and Suicide Support do tremendous work. However, still too many people slip through the cracks. Dementia through alcohol and drug abuse is on the rise. Pot smoking, LSD licking, heroin injecting and the use of a plethora of different drugs are on the rise. Violence is on the rise with it. Long Term Care facilities await the onslaught of those who abuse their bodies and brains.

To date, there are only 2,257 beds available for a population of 253,000. I fear it is nowhere near enough. People are queuing up to join the list, trying to get into these scarce few beds. At the moment, there is no answer to the upcoming crisis. The government seems to be wearing blinkers when confronting the issue. What do those in power see?

The Saskatoon Health Regional Authority serves 342,362 people (as of 2014 SHRA report). This includes one hundred cities, towns, villages, Rural Municipalities and Native communities. There are seventy-five facilities, of which nine are hospitals (three, St. Paul's, Royal University and City Hospital are tertiary with each of those in Saskatoon.) There are thirty long-term care facilities.

The Health Region employs 1036 physicians: 14,145 health care providers, support staff and managers. There are also 6,010 volunteers. The total area of the health care region is 34,120 square kilometres.

The previous CEO of the Saskatoon Health Region received more than $400,000/year in wages and benefits. We should, perhaps, put this wage into perspective. The Prime Minister of Canada receives an annual salary of $260,000 while the Chancellor of Germany received an annual salary of $234,000. The President of the United States earns a salary of $400,000. (All salaries are in Canadian Dollars and are as of 2014).

Things seem a little topsy-turvy. The Chancellor of Germany has the health, welfare and safety of eighty-three million people. The President of the United States likewise has responsibilities for 315 million people and, perhaps, the safety and security of the free-speaking world. And of course, our own Prime Minister, who is responsible for thirty-five million Canadians. $400,000 for taking care of a paltry 343,362 people seems a little excessive. But then it becomes worse. The union leader of SEIU West received a salary of $94,000 to care for a Unionist workforce of approximately 12,000 members. And union dues? Between six and seven hundred dollars a year for a CCA.

THE SURVEYS

A 2014 survey of long-term care posed this question to family members:

Having trust in the staff is also very important. How would you rate your satisfaction with the staff's professionalism, competence, knowledge, and ability to provide excellent care?

A full twenty-two percent replied with either neutral or negative response. The high number, I believe, reflects the Health Region and the union's position in allowing long-term care facilities to hire incompetent, untrained care aides.

It is permissible to use untrained Care aides. The only restriction? They must, within two years, gain their diploma. These people are trained by regular staff to perform often complex, dangerous tasks. Rarely do we find regular staff having teaching credentials. There is no syllabus to follow, no teaching plan and no follow-up by any professional instructor. The new Care Aide will often be trained by a variety of staff with some of them incompetent in their skills.

This absurd policy is sanctioned by both the SEIU West and SHRA. One has to ask whether we have the resident's welfare at heart, or are we more interested in relieving the pressure of short staffing of professional care aides, or perhaps in a swelling of union coffers? Whatever the case, these untrained people are entering a workplace that requires a high degree of skills. Knowledge of illnesses and communication skills are essential. And yet we allow people with little or no knowledge to enter this profession. It is not uncommon for these untrained people to be burdened with language difficulties, making the task of the so-called trainers even more difficult. It is, without a doubt, a farce of epic proportions, and it must be stopped.

It is interesting to note that untrained Care Aides will immediately gain seniority hours. This will enable them to bid on posted positions within the health district. They will also collect the standard rate of pay all Care Aides receive. Meanwhile, their educated colleague who worked hard in school to achieve academic standards will not begin to accrue seniority until they find employment. Unlike their untrained counterparts, they will discover that when they enter the workforce, they have been penalised. They will not have received any income or seniority when they were in school. It has happened where a new grad CCA, who possesses all the skills necessary to complete assigned tasks, will lose a posted position to an untrained colleague because they do not have sufficient seniority. It is a dangerous practice. Injustice, it seems, occurs around every corner.

From the survey of a different facility:

Having trust in the staff is also very important. How would you rate your satisfaction with the staff's professionalism, competence, knowledge, and ability to provide excellent care?

With this question, eighteen percent were either neutral or negative with their response.

Timeliness of communication about changes in your care needs?

They answered with an astounding **forty-five percent** either neutral or negative response. One can only conclude that either staff were busy and didn't have time to communicate with residents; that staff didn't feel the need, or that staff felt the resident would not understand. Therefore, changes were made arbitrarily.

Feeling Listened to?

Twenty-seven percent replied that they felt they were not being listened to. A full thirty percent of family members answered the same question either neutral or negative responses. The answer to the previous question applies

Have you reported any concerns to the staff in the past year?

Family members returned an astonishing sixty-nine percent as yes.

Residents Taking Concerns to Management. How many times have you been dissatisfied with how a concern was addressed and then taken to management?

1-2: 35%

3-4: 9%

5-6: 5%

*Do you feel confident that you will **not** suffer because of having raised concerns?*

A full thirty-five percent felt that they would suffer because of filing a complaint. As a Care Aide, the answers bother me. Why would anyone suffer because of complaining to management? Could it be that this is where true abuse lay? Is the abuse intended to stop the resident from going forward again? Are other staff members behaving in an irrational way by continuing the abusive care to support a troublesome colleague? I trust not, but it appears to be all for one and one for all.

What of the availability of care team members (special care aides, nurses, doctors, therapists)? Thirty-two percent of residents responded with either neutral or negative while family members responded with a full forty percent either neutral or negative. The high number of neutral or negative response numbers exasperate me for I have been vocal with anyone who will listen that staffing levels are low. In Long Term Care facilities, they are kept deliberately low.

THE NEXT-TO-LAST WORD

Cases of abuse; Cases of neglect; Cases of misconduct; Cases where action could have been taken to avoid the continual wrongdoing; Cases resulting in the indignity to human life; Cases of inhumane treatment that could have been avoided.

I came forward explaining the above, seeking only to right the wrong being done. I came forward revealing that the wrongdoings were a fault of the system and not of the worker. I came forward stating that this abuse was caused by a shortage of staff and nothing else. I believed through the exhaustive interrogation process that the point had been proven.

I came forward stating that residents were in their night pads from six to twelve hours and many were not turned or changed for that amount of time. During the investigation, I had no trouble in providing circumstantial evidence of residents in bed and not being turned for up to ten hours. As for twelve hours? That proved a little more difficult. But the truth, as always, was just around the next corner.

LIFE GOES ON

It took time, a long time, too long really. But in the end a rose remained a rose, CEO's remained defiant, and politicians continued to be politicians. The CEO's of the Saskatoon Health Region Authority and at my employ remained at their post. All the players continued with their respective roles. No one had disturbed the playing field. Nothing had changed.

It was a waste of my time, the CEO's time, the politicians' time. It was a waste of taxpayers' money (I do not know how much the investigation cost. I probably never will, and I suspect the taxpayer never will either). And, of course, it was a waste of the publics time.

The costs should have been negligible, buried in a typical workday. But politicians always try to make political hay out of peoples' lives. That's what they do. Never do we see a politician stand and speak without some direct, or indirect, reference to the people they are supposed to serve. If I sound cynical, I am, with gusto and verve.

I am about to lead you into the quagmire of what transpired after the investigation had concluded. I think it fair to the reader to understand what the Saskatchewan government did to absolve itself of the political mess in which it had buried itself.

The Union (SEIU West) was more than happy to take the matter of my termination to arbitration. I had several visits with the union solicitors at the union office. The three of us -- the union chief bargainer, the solicitor, and myself -- first sat down in the early fall of 2015 to discuss possible arbitration. At the same time, I had retained a lawyer to litigate against the provincial government for their biased and, what I thought, illegal release of my private and confidential information to the public.

My case never went to arbitration. An agreement was reached. There was an apparent reason why the parties reached a settlement. Eight days had been put aside for the hearing. Later another five were added, just in case they were needed. A panel of three arbitrators was slated to hear the case in July of 2015. The cost of such action would have been more than I would have earned in almost three years. My employer would have borne half of the expenses. The other half, of course, fell to the Union. Both sides would have to bear the responsibility of fifty percent of all costs, which, in arbitration, are rarely awarded.

When presented with the final settlement, it was evident the Provincial government, Saskatchewan Health and my employer would not allow me to inform anyone of the settlement. I was muzzled. No one was to know the outcome of financial gain if there was any. I accepted that without reservation. To say my lips are sealed is an understatement.

There is, of course, more. In my letter of termination, accusations of some of the most unspeakable acts against my residents were laid against me by my colleagues. Allegations of physical abuse to residents, racism towards staff, harassment of staff, posting derogatory remarks about staff and management on social media, refusing direction from a supervisor, etc.

It was made clear during the investigation none of the allegations had been proven, that all were facetious, innuendo, falsehoods. I discovered that the lead investigator had attempted to solicit other ills against me. The investigator alluded to this during the investigation, belittling both my union rep and myself for our accusation against him. Not only did I discover the truth, but the Care Aide in question was also the only complainant not issued a subpoena to attend the hearing.

The cover-up was complete. My employer failed to do their duty and to report my concerns to their superiors. Discovering my complaints led the Saskatoon Health Region Authority to release private and confidential information without my approval. They then sent my file to Saskatchewan Health who in turn sent it to the Communications Director of the Saskatchewan Party (the government). She then distributed some of the information to the media. Either purposefully or inadvertently, she sent some half-truths and non-truths to the press.

Management had made a terrible mistake. SHRA had made a major blunder, Saskatchewan Health had made a colossal error in judgment, and the Premier had destroyed my working life.

When I signed the memorandum of agreement, my termination was corrected (amongst other things). My record of employment would now show as being laid off. The fact that my expertise with dementia residents was sorely needed, that there was a chronic shortage of Continuing Care Aides, meant nothing. I was sent out into the wilderness with sorely needed skills. That wilderness is called a blacklist.

At my termination meeting of August 13, 2014, I was made aware that under no circumstances would I ever work for SHRA or its affiliates. I could apply for work, but that was as far as my application would go. I was informed that I would not be allowed to enter my workplace. When questioned about the possibility of having a family member living in the facility, my employer said that it would not preclude me from being removed should I attempt to visit that person.

After being questioned by my union rep, clarity was not forthcoming. My employer had muddied the waters. It was clear he had put his foot in his mouth without any thought of the consequences. Without a definite answer from my ex-employer, and in writing, it is feasible I could have a family member living in that facility, and I would not be able to visit them. The word "disgust" reverberates.

The Office of the Independent Privacy Commission's report strongly suggested I receive an apology.

I have duly received apologies from the CEO of SHRA, and from Saskatchewan Health, both in written form. I also received a very public verbal apology from the Premier while he was at a press conference in the Legislature rotunda. However, I have never received an apology from my employer or anyone connected with that Long-Term Care facility. My co-workers have never apologised for their behaviour toward me.

I have concluded my employer believes they are of loftier heights than that of the Premier and his cabinet. I have come to believe the CEO to be an incredibly arrogant, almost narcissistic, man.

Whistleblowers, to a fault, never win. Employment becomes a thing of the past. Families face the torture of being ripped apart. Some have faced arrest, and some can never find their way back to normalcy. Suicide is sometimes the final solution.

I cannot work in Saskatchewan. I had placed over eighty applications with just one response. I, therefore, have spent my time becoming an on-line healthcare critic. I will not rest until Saskatchewan Health realises its critical role in our society.

The people of Saskatchewan deserve better. The Elderly deserve not only proper care but also respect, something that is sadly lacking.

I am content with the work I have done. I am proud of my ability to care for the elderly that reside in Long-Term Care facilities. I am equally honoured to have made a difference in people's lives.

See Me

What do you see, nurses, what do you see?
Are you thinking, when you look at me –
A crabby old woman, not very wise,
Uncertain of habit, with far-away eyes,
Who dribbles her food and makes no reply,
When you say in a loud voice — "I do wish you'd try."

Who seems not to notice the things that you do,
And forever is losing a stocking or shoe,
Who unresisting or not, lets you do as you will,
With bathing and feeding, the long day to fill.
Is that what you're thinking, is that what you see?

Then open your eyes, nurse, you're looking at ME…
I'll tell you who I am, as I sit here so still;
As I rise at your bidding, as I eat at your will.

I'm a small child of ten with a father and mother,
Brothers and sisters, who love one another,
A young girl of sixteen with wings on her feet.
Dreaming that soon now a lover she'll meet;
A bride soon at twenty — my heart gives a leap,
Remembering the vows that I promised to keep;

At twenty-five now I have young of my own,
Who need me to build a secure, happy home;
A woman of thirty, my young now grow fast,
Bound to each other with ties that should last;

At forty, my young sons have grown and are gone,
But my man's beside me to see I don't mourn;
At fifty once more babies play 'round my knee,
Again we know children, my loved one and me.

Dark days are upon me, my husband is dead,
I look at the future, I shudder with dread,
For my young are all rearing young of their own,
And I think of the years and the love that I've known;
I'm an old woman now and nature is cruel –
'Tis her jest to make old age look like a fool.

The body is crumbled, grace and vigour depart,
There is now a stone where once I had a heart,
But inside this old carcas a young girl still dwells,
And now and again my battered heart swells.

I remember the joys, I remember the pain,
And I'm loving and living life over again,
I think of the years, all too few — gone too fast,
And accept the stark fact that nothing can last –
So I open your eyes, nurses, open and see,
Not a crabby old woman, look closer, nurses — see ME!

This poem was found among the possessions of an elderly lady who died in the geriatric ward of a hospital. No information is available concerning her — who she was or when she died. Reprinted from the "Assessment and Alternatives Help Guide" prepared by the Colorado Foundation for Medical Care.

www.ingramcontent.com/pod-product-compliance
Lightning Source LLC
Chambersburg PA
CBHW071420180526
45170CB00001B/160